Milady's
Human Anatomy
& Physiology
Workbook

Milady's Human Anatomy & Physiology Workbook

Maura T. Scali-Sheahan

Milady Publishing Company
(A Division of Delmar Publishers Inc.)

NOTICE TO THE READER

Cover: design by Nicole Reamer

Milady Staff
Publisher: Catherine Frangie
Senior Project Editor: Laura V. Miller
Production Manager: John Mickelbank
Sr. Art Design/Supervisor: Susan Mathews

Freelance Developmental Editor: Pamela Fuller

For information address:
Milady Publishing Company
(A Division of Delmar Publishers Inc.)
3 Columbia Circle, Box 12519
Albany, NY 12212-2519

Printed in the United States of America
Printed and distributed simultaneously in Canada

1 2 3 4 5 6 7 8 9 10 XXX 00 99 98 97 96 95 94 93

Library of Congress Cataloging-in-Publication Data
Scali-Sheahan, Maura T.
    Milady's human anatomy & physiology workbook / Maura T. Scali-Sheahan.
        p.   cm.
    Includes index.
    ISBN 1-56253-157-3
    1. Human anatomy. 2. Human physiology. 3. Beauty operators.
    I. Title. II. Title: Milady's human anatomy & physiology workbook.
QM23.2.S28   1994
612—dc20   93-45428
                                                  CIP

ISBN 1-56253-157-3

Contents

Acknowledgments   ix
Introduction   xi

Chapter 1
The Body as a Whole   1
The Study of Anatomy   1
Anatomical Terms   2
Cavities of the Body   2
Life Functions   4
Human Development   4
Chemistry   5
   Elements   6
   Compounds   7
   Acids, Bases, and Salts   9
   Potential Hydrogen (pH)   10
The Cell   10
   Movement of Materials Across Cell Membranes   13
   Specialization   16
Tissues   21
   Organs and Systems   22
   Tissue Repair   22
Integumentary System   23
   Structure of the Skin   24
   Appendages of the Skin   26
The Skin and Its Relationship to Bacteria   28
Review   31

Chapter 2
Physiology and Histology of the Hair   37
Follicle Formation   37
   Primary Hair   37
   Secondary Hair   38
   Tertiary Hair   38
Structure of the Follicle   39
   Hair Root   41
   Other Structures Connected with the Follicle   42
   Sudoriferous (Sweat) Glands   42
The Structure of the Hair   42
   The Cuticle   42

The Cortex   43
How the Cortex and the Cuticle Work Together   45
Medulla   46
Hair Growth and the Nature of Protein   46
  Bonds of the Hair Cortex   48
Formation of Hard Keratin in Hair   49
  Anagen Stage   49
  Mature Hair Fiber   50
  Catagen Phase   51
  Telogen   51
Review   53

Chapter 3

The Body Framework   **59**
Introduction to the Skeletal System   59
Bone Types   59
Joints   59
Types of Motion   61
Structure and Formation of Bone   61
  Bone Formation   62
  Structure   62
Parts of the Skeleton   63
  Axial Skeleton   63
  Appendicular Skeleton   66
Disorders of the Bones and Joints   69
  Common Types of Fractures   69
  Bone and Joint Injuries   69
Review   71

Chapter 4

The Muscular System   **75**
Types of Muscles   75
Attachment of Muscles   75
Physiotherapy   79
  Classification of Massage Movements   82
  Basic Scalp Massage   83
Musculoskeletal Disorders   85
The Effects of Massage   88
Review   91

Chapter 5

Transport of Blood and Oxygen   **95**
Functions of Blood   95
Major Blood Circuits   97
The Heart   98

Structure of the Heart 98
Function and Path of General Circulation 100
Blood Pressure 103
Pulse 104
The Blood 104
Blood Plasma 105
Red Blood Cells 106
White Blood Cells 106
Blood Platelets 106
Blood Types 107
RH Factor 107
The Lymphatic System and Immunity 107
Natural and Acquired Immunities 108
Hypersensitivity 108
Disorders of the Circulatory System 109
Disorders of the Heart 109
Disorders of the Blood Vessels 110
Disorders of the Blood 110
AIDS 111
The Stages of AIDS 112
Preventing AIDS 112
Review 115

Chapter 6
The Respiratory System 121
Respiratory Organs and Structures 122
Nasal Cavity 122
The Pharynx 122
The Larynx 122
The Trachea 124
The Bronchi, Bronchioles, and Alveoli 124
The Lungs 124
Mechanics of Breathing 125
Respiratory Disorders 126
Review 129

Chapter 7
The Digestive System 133
The Role of Nutrients 135
Water 135
Carbohydrates 135
Lipids 135
Proteins 135
Vitamins 136
Minerals 136

Dietary Guidelines   139
Foods and Food Processing   141
Eating Disorders   142
Disorders of the Digestive System   143
Review   147

Chapter 8
The Elimination of Waste   151
The Excretory System   151
    The Urinary Tract   151
Disorders of the Excretory System   152
Review   155

Chapter 9
Regulators of Body Functions   157
The Endocrine System   157
    The Pituitary Gland   157
    Other Glands   157
Disorders of the Endocrine System   159
    Pituitary Disorders   160
    Adrenal Disorders   160
Review   161

Chapter 10
The Nervous System   163
Central Nervous System   164
The Reflex Act   165
Disorders of the Nervous System   166
Disorders of the Sense Organs   167
    Ear Disorders   167
    Eye Disorders   167
Review   169

Bibliography   173
Glossary/Index   175
Answers to Review Questions   189

Acknowledgments

I would like to personally thank the authors of the texts mentioned in the bibliography of this book. I compliment you all on your thoroughness and dedication to your chosen areas of expertise and hope that I have made good use of a mere fraction of that valuable information. As always, it can be difficult to separate the essential from the interesting when there is so much good material from which to draw!

Of course, I want to thank Catherine Frangie, editor extraordinaire, for challenging me once again with an exciting project!

I dedicate this work in loving memory of my father, who is still a constant source of inspiration for all things creative, and to my mother who, when the challenges of life aren't sufficient, promptly designs one of her own!

Last, but certainly not least, I would like to thank my children, Nathan, Sarah, and Rachel, for putting up with "something easy" dinners and pizza for the duration of this project—thanks, kids.

Introduction

Welcome to our latest multifaceted creation, *Milady's Human Anatomy & Physiology Workbook!*

This text has been prepared to supplement the full array of Milady's beauty industry publications, from *Milady's Standard Textbook of Cosmetology* to *Modern Esthetics* and *The Theory and Practice of Therapeutic Massage.*

The *Human Anatomy & Physiology Workbook* provides detailed descriptions and explanations of the structures, functions, and interrelated processes of the human body. Most important, it strives to highlight those areas of knowledge that are of particular interest to the beauty care professional and applicable to the performance of services on clients.

Each chapter is formatted to present the subject matter, applied theory, and chapter review tests as a workbook to enhance your knowledge, understanding, and professionalism. It also provides the professional with an excellent source of reference material that goes beyond certain areas within our specialized texts without being overtly oriented to the medical profession.

"The Body as a Whole," Chapter 1, provides you with an overview of the body and its systems and structures. Special attention is given to the integumentary system because it is such a vital component in the performance of client services.

Chapter 2, "Physiology and Histology of the Hair," is another specific area of concern for people in the beauty care industry, and every effort has been made to provide detailed information from a variety of sources and applicable theory.

Chapter 3, "The Body Framework" covers the skeletal system, including its functions and characteristics.

The muscular system is discussed in Chapter 4, with special emphasis on the methods and effects of massage.

Chapter 5, provides an in-depth look at the transport of blood and oxygen, which is all-important to the condition of the skin, hair, scalp, and nails.

Chapter 6 explains the breathing process in detail and offers the causes and symptoms of many respiratory disorders, some of which we may experience in the shop or salon.

From the most minute cell structure to nutritional guidelines, "The Digestive System," Chapter 7, explores in detail the processes, functions, and effects of this important system.

In Chapter 8, we examine the excretory system and the elimination of waste.

"Regulators of Body Functions," Chapter 9, concerns the endocrine glands and reviews their functions and interactions within the human body system.

In Chapter 10, the components of the nervous system are discussed, including the function of the brain.

It is hoped that this text will prove to be of value to students, licensed professionals, and instructors as a resource to be used again and again. For the student, this text offers additional insight into the workings of the human body that may not be covered in your specialized texts. This is especially true of disorders and conditions that you had no prior knowledge of but may now be able to recognize because you have encountered them through working with clients.

For the licensed professional, this text serves as an excellent reminder of the interrelationship and interdependence of all the body's systems and of your role in performing services that harmonize with them. It also serves as a reference source that any professional working within any of the specialized fields within our industry should find helpful. You may even end up sharing a lot of what you learn from this volume with your clients during the course of conversation while performing services!

For the instructor, this text provides the "auxiliary" text you've been waiting for, both in the classroom as an additional workbook and/or for your own supplemental material to curricula. Many instructors encounter students who always want to know more or require a more detailed explanation of the "how and why" of things in order to appease their learning curiosity. This text provides you with a learning tool to help you and your students to achieve these goals.

On a final note, a number of sources were used for the compilation of this text. These are listed in the bibliography. It is recommended that you seek out these references for more detailed information on a specific topic or field of the beauty care industry.

1

The Body as a Whole

Anatomy and physiology are branches of a larger science called biology, which is the study of all forms of life.

Anatomy is the study of the shape and structure of an organism's body and the relationship of one body part to another.

Physiology studies the function of each body part and how these functions coordinate to form a complete living organism.

The Study of Anatomy

Anatomy is divided into many branches based on the investigative technique used, the type of knowledge to be sought, or the parts of the body under study.

Gross anatomy is the study of large and easily observable structures of an organism. It is done through dissection or inspection with the naked eye. Different body parts and regions are studied with regard to their general shape, external features, and main divisions.

> *The beauty care professional practices a form of gross anatomical study when in the process of analyzing facial features for hair design or makeup application, and dermatology when performing skin analysis for facials or examining the condition of nails for manicures or pedicures.*

Microscopic anatomy is a branch of anatomy that is further subdivided into two types—**cytology (seye-TAWL-oh-jee)**, the study of the structure, function, and development of cells that make up different body parts, and **histology**, which studies the tissues and organs making up the entire body of an organism.

Developmental anatomy studies the growth and development of a organism during its lifetime.

Comparative anatomy is the study of the different body parts and organs of humans with regard to the similarities and differences to other animals in the animal kingdom.

Systemic (sis-TEM-ik) anatomy is the study of the structure and function of various organs or parts making up a particular organ system. Systemic anatomy is further subdivided to include:

Angiology (an-jee-AWL-ohjee)—study of the circulatory system.

Arthrology—study of the joints.

Dermatology—study of the integumentary system (skin, hair and nails).

1

Endocrinology (en-doh-krin-AWL-oh-jee)—study of the endocrine, or hormonal, system.

Myology (meye-AWL-oh-jee)—study of the muscular system.

Neurology (ner-AWL-oh-jee)—study of the nervous system.

Osteology (oss-tee-AWL-oh-jee)—study of the skeletal system.

Splanchnology (splank-NAWL-oh-jee)—collective study of the digestive, respiratory, reproductive, and urinary systems.

> *Although the beauty care professional will most often deal with the integumentary system, a basic study of angiology, arthrology, myology, and neurology is of vital importance when performing any type of massage treatment to the scalp, face, neck, hands, or feet.*

Anatomical Terms

In the study of anatomy and physiology, specific terms are used to describe either the specific location of a structure or organ or the relative position of one body part to another. The following anatomical terminology is used to describe the human body as it is standing in what is known as the anatomical position (simply, the person stands erect, face forward, arms at sides, and palms forward).

Term	Meaning
Anterior (ventral	front.
Ventral	in front of.
Posterior (dorsal)	back.
Dorsal	in back of.
Cranial (superior)	head end of body (refers to direction).
Caudal	tail end of body (refers to direction).
Superior	upper, or above another.
Inferior (caudal)	lower, or below another.
Medial (sagittal)	toward the midline plane of the body.
Lateral	away, or toward the side of the body.
Proximal	toward the point of attachment to the body.
Distal	away from the point of attachment or origin.
Superficial	on or near the surface.
Internal	involving an internal organ or structure.

> *The above anatomical terminology may prove to be of value to the professional during the client consultation when discussing health conditions or when reading a physician's recommendation or prescription directions. (See Figure 1–1.)*

Cavities of the Body

The organs that comprise most of the nine body systems are organized into several cavities: the cranial, spinal, thoracic, and abdominopelvic. These cavities fit into two

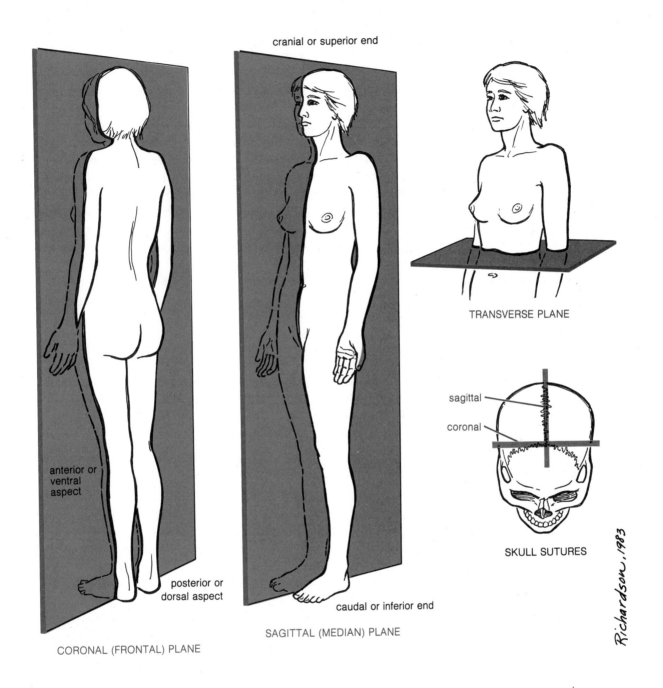

Figure 1-1 Anatomical terms are used to describe body divisions.

larger cavities, the dorsal and ventral cavities. The cranial and spinal cavities are within the larger dorsal cavity, and the thoracic and abdominopelvic cavities are found in the ventral cavity region. The dorsal and ventral cavities make up the two major body cavities. (See Figure 1–2.)

> *Of special note to the professional are the smaller cavities located within the anterior cranial region, which include the orbital, nasal, and buccal cavities. The nerves and muscles associated with these areas are highly influenced by massage, pressure, steam, light, and the immediate environment. The professional should be conscious of effects that may be caused by any of these factors, such as, under- or overstimulation in massage; the correct use of different types of pressure on the skin and its underlying structure; the effects of steam, especially as it relates to sinus and nasal cavities; light and its penetration abilities; and the negative or positive effect of the environment, especially odors or scents. Odors originating from perm solutions or other chemicals may cause allergic reactions when inhaled or, conversely, aroma therapy may be used during facial or body massages for inducing a more harmonious inner balance.*

Life Functions

Life functions are a series of highly organized and related activities that are vital to the life, growth, and maintenance of living organisms. Vital life functions include movement, ingestion, digestion, transport, respiration, synthesis, assimilation, growth, secretion, excretion, regulation and reproduction. (See Table 1–1.)

Human Development

Each of us inherits a range of size, a form, and a life span through the gametes (sperm and egg cells) from our parents. Living depends on the constant release of energy, derived from food, in every cell of the body. Powered thus, cells are able to maintain their own functions and living conditions.

Early in human development, certain groups of cells become highly specialized for specific functions, such as motion or response.

Tissues are special cells grouped according to function, shape, size, and structure. Tissues form larger functional and structural units known as organs. A good example is human skin, which is an organ composed of epithelial, connective, muscular, and nervous tissue.

Metabolism (meh-TAH-boh-lis-em) is the sum of all the chemical reactions within a cell, including functional activities, which result in growth, repair, energy release, the use of food, and secretions. Metabolism consists of two opposite processes: anabolism and catabolism. Anabolism is the building up of complex materials from simpler ones, while catabolism is the breaking down and changing of complex substances into simpler ones, with an accompanying release of energy.

The **organs** of the body function interdependently with one another to form a whole, live, functioning organism. Many organs are grouped together because they perform a related function, such as digestion; these are known as organ systems. The

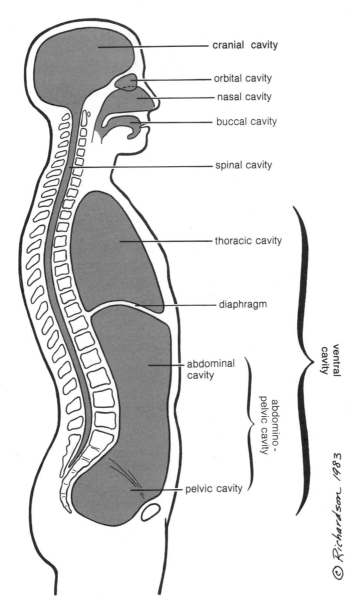

cranial cavity

orbital cavity

nasal cavity

buccal cavity

spinal cavity

thoracic cavity

diaphragm

abdominal cavity

abdomino-pelvic cavity

ventral cavity

pelvic cavity

© Richardson 1983

Figure 1-2   Cavities of the body

functioning of a complex organism, such as the human body, requires the combined activities of cells, tissues, organs, and systems.

Chemistry

Chemistry is the study of the structure of matter—the composition of substances, their properties, and their chemical reactions and synthesis. Chemical reactions within the human body take place continually, from the digestion of food to the manufacture of proteins in a single cell. In fact, it is in the chemical reactions within cells that the necessities to sustain life occur. This study of the chemical reactions within living things is known as biochemistry.

Table 1-1   Review of the Life Functions

LIFE FUNCTIONS	DEFINITION
Movement	The ability of the whole organism – or a part of it – to move
Ingestion	The process by which an organism takes in food
Digestion	The breakdown of complex food molecules into simpler food molecules
Transport	The movement of necessary substances to, into, and around cells, and of cellular products and wastes out and away from cells
Respiration	The burning or oxidation of food molecules in a cell to release energy, water and carbon dioxide
Synthesis	The combination of simple molecules into more complex molecules to help an organism build new tissue
Assimilation	The transformation of digested food molecules into living tissue for growth and self-repair
Growth	The enlargment of an organism due to synthesis and assimilation, resulting in an increase in the number and size of its cells
Secretion	The formation and release of substances from a cell or structure
Excretion	The removal of metabolic waste products from an organism
Regulation (sensitivity)	The ability of an organism to respond to its environment so as to maintain a balanced state (homeostasis)
Reproduction	The ability of an organism to produce offspring with similar characteristics. This is *essential* for species survival as opposed to individual survival

Elements

Matter can exist in one of three states or phases—solid, liquid, or gas. Nonliving matter may exist in only one phase however, while although living matter may appear solid, it usually contains more than one phase. In the case of the human body, bone matter is basically solid, body fluid is basically liquid, and the contents of the lungs are basically gaseous.

When matter is broken down into its smallest basic particles, it is found that these particles are the same. These are the basic building blocks of all matter and are known as elements. An **element (El-eh-ment)** is a substance in its simplest form: it cannot be broken down any further by usual means. There are 92 natural elements which are found in nature, and at least 13 man-made elements. Twenty of the 105 elements are found in all living things, and among the 20 are 4 elements that make up 97 percent of all living matter—carbon, oxygen, hydrogen, and nitrogen.

Elements in Living Matter

Carbon	C
Oxygen	O
Hydrogen	H
Nitrogen	N
Sodium	Na
Chlorine	Cl
Magnesium	Mg
Phosphorous	P
Sulfur	S
Calcium	Ca
Potassium	K

Trace Elements

Iron	Fe
Copper	Cu
Manganese	Mn
Zinc	Zn
Boron	B
Tin	Sn
Vanadium	V
Cobalt	Co
Molybdenum	Mo

Compounds

When elements combine together in a definite proportion by weight, compounds are formed. A compound has different characteristics or properties from the elements of which the compound is composed. For example, water (H_2O) is a compound that consists of two parts of hydrogen and one part of oxygen. Separately, hydrogen and oxygen are gaseous elements, but when combined together to form water, the result is a liquid compound.

Just as elements are represented by symbols, compounds are represented by formulas. A formula shows the types of elements present and the proportion of each element by weight.

Molecules A molecule is the smallest unit of a compound that still has the properties of the compound and has the ability to lead its own stable and independent existence.

Again using the example of water, the compound water can be broken down into the smallest unit and still retain the molecule water, H_2O.

Types of Compounds   All known compounds can be classified into two groups—inorganic and organic compounds.

Inorganic compounds are generally compounds that do not contain the element carbon. The two exceptions are carbon dioxide and calcium carbonate.

Organic compounds always contain the element carbon combined with hydrogen and other elements. They are found in living things and in the substances that they produce. The four main groups of organic compounds are carbohydrates, lipids, proteins, and nucleic acids.

Carbohydrates   All carbohydrates are compounds composed of the elements carbon, hydrogen, and oxygen and are further divided into three groups—monosaccharides, disaccharides, and polysaccharides.

Monosaccharides (mon-oh-SAK-ah-reyeds) are single or simple sugars which cannot be broken down further, such as glucose, fructose, and galactose. Glucose (also called blood sugar) is carried by the bloodstream and is the main source of energy in the cells.

Disaccharides (deye-SAK-ah-reyeds) are formed by two monosaccharide molecules and are known as double sugars. Examples include sucrose (table sugar), maltose (malt sugar), and lactose (milk sugar).

Polysaccharides are found in, or made by, living organisms and microbes and consist of glucose molecules bonded together in a chain-like fashion. Examples are starch, cellulose, and glycogen.

Lipids   Lipids are molecules containing the elements carbon, hydrogen, and oxygen. They differ from carbohydrates in having a lesser amount of oxygen relative to hydrogen. Lipids include fats, oils, and waxes.

Proteins   Proteins are among the most essential organic compounds found in all living organisms. They are composed of carbon, hydrogen, oxygen, nitrogen, and, most often, phosphorous and sulfur. Proteins are found in every part of a living cell and serve as the binding and structural components of all living things. Protein is a larger molecule composed of smaller molecular units called amino acids.

Table 1–2   The Nine Essential Amino Acids

ESSENTIAL AMINO ACIDS	SYMBOL
Histidine	His
Isoleucine	Ileu
Leucine	Leu
Lysine	Lys
Methionine	Met
Phenylalanine	Phe
Threonine	Trp
Tryptophan	Try
Valine	Val

Table 1-3 Name, Formula, Location, and Use of Some Common Acids

NAME OF ACID	FORMULA	WHERE FOUND OR USAGE
Acetic acid	CH_3COOH	Found in vinegar
Boric acid	H_3BO_3	Weak eyewash
Carbonic acid	H_2CO_3	Found in carbonated beverages
Hydrochloric acid	HCl	Found in stomach
Nitric acid	HNO_3	Industrial oxidizing acid
Sulfuric acid	H_2SO_4	Found in batteries and industrial mineral acid

Table 1–2 lists the nine essential amino acids that must be ingested because the body cannot produce them.

Enzymes Enzymes are specialized protein molecules found in all living cells and help control the various chemical reactions occurring within them. Although an enzyme affects the rate or speed of a chemical reaction, it does so without itself being changed.

Nucleic Acids (noo-KLAY-ik) Nucleic acids are essential organic compounds containing the elements carbon, oxygen, hydrogen, nitrogen, and phosphorous. The two types of nucleic acids are DNA, which is involved in the heredity process, and RNA, which is essential in helping cells to synthesize proteins.

Acids, Bases, and Salts

An **acid** is a substance that, when dissolved in water, will ionize (separate into either positively or negatively charged particles when in a solution) into positively charged hydrogen ions and negatively charged ions of some other element. (See Table 1–3.)

A **base** or alkali is a substance that, when dissolved in water, ionizes into negatively charged hydroxide ions and positively charged ions of a metal. (See Table 1–4.)

When an acid and a base are combined, they form a **salt** plus water, causing a reaction known as neutralization. In the neutralization reaction, hydrogen ions from

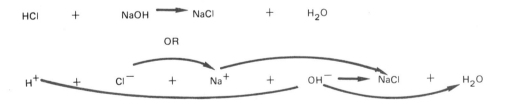

Figure 1-3 The neutralization reaction

Table 1-4 Name, Formula, Location, and Use of Some Common Bases

NAME OF BASE	FORMULA	WHERE FOUND OR USAGE
Ammonium hydroxide	NH_4OH	Household liquid cleaners
Magnesium hydroxide	$Mg(OH)_2$	Milk of magnesia
Potassium hydroxide	KOH	Caustic potash
Sodium hydroxide	NaOH	Lye

the acid and hydroxide ions from the base join to form water, while at the same time, the negative ions of the acid combine with positive ions from the base to form the compound salt. (See Figure 1–3.)

Potential Hydrogen (pH)

Potential hydrogen (pH) is the measure of the **acidity** (hydrogen ions) or **alkalinity** (hydroxide ions) of a solution. The pH scale measures the acidity or alkalinity of a solution with a range of 0 to 14. A pH of 7 indicates that there are the same number of hydrogen ions as hydroxide ions in a solution and constitutes a neutral pH. (Pure water has a neutral pH.) A pH value of 4 is ten times as acidic as a pH of 5; the lower the pH number, the greater the hydrogen ion concentration. A pH value of 9 is ten times as alkaline, or higher in hydroxide ions, as a pH of 8. (See Figure 1–4.)

In order for living cells to function properly, their biochemical reactions must occur at a given pH. In humans and other living organisms, the maintenance of a balanced pH—where fluids are neither too acidic nor too basic (alkaline)—is achieved through a compound called a buffer. Sodium bicarbonate is one such buffer, which is often used to neutralize or balance the gastric juices of an upset stomach.

> *Many terms and definitions have been presented in the foregoing information with which the professional may or may not be familiar. A basic understanding of chemistry is essential for the professional due to the nature of the products used in the beauty care industry. We find the terms* amino acids *and* nucleic acids *used in many hair and skin products, and therefore, we should possess some understanding of the function or properties of these ingredients and whether they can make a difference in the results of our client service.*

The Cell

The cell is the basic unit of structure and function of all living things. A cell is surrounded by a cell membrane, and each cell has a unique function. The **cell membrane** separates the cell's cytoplasm from its external environment and from neighboring cells. In addition, it regulates the passage of certain molecules into and out of the cell, letting in some while preventing the passage of others. The cell membrane is made of protein and lipid (fatty substance) molecules arranged in a layered design, with the lipids in the middle between two layers of protein. (See Figure 1–5.)

The **cytoplasm (SEYE-toh-plaz-em)** is a sticky, semifluid substance found between the nucleus and the cell membrane. It consists of proteins, lipids, carbohydrates, minerals, salts, and water (70–90 percent). The substances vary from one cell and/or organism to the next. The cytoplasm is the background for all the chemical reactions within a cell, including protein synthesis and cell respiration. The cytoplasm moves in a circular motion, transporting molecules throughout the cell. It houses **organelles (or-gan-ElS)** (cell structures) that help the cell to function. These are the nucleus, mitochondria, ribosomes, Golgi apparatus, endoplasmic reticulum, and lysosomes.

The most important organelle within the cell is the **nucleus (NOO-klee-us)**, which has two vital functions: to control the activities of the cell and to facilitate cell division. The nucleus is located in or near the cell's center and contains DNA and protein.

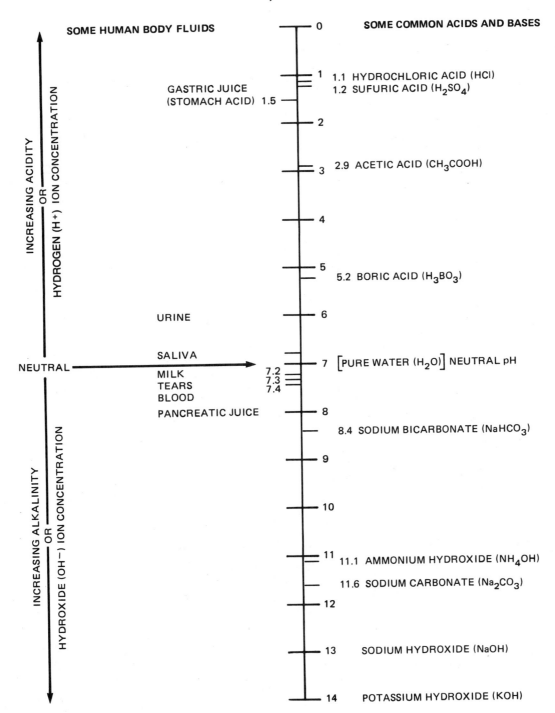

Figure 1-4   pH values of some common acids, bases, and human body fluids

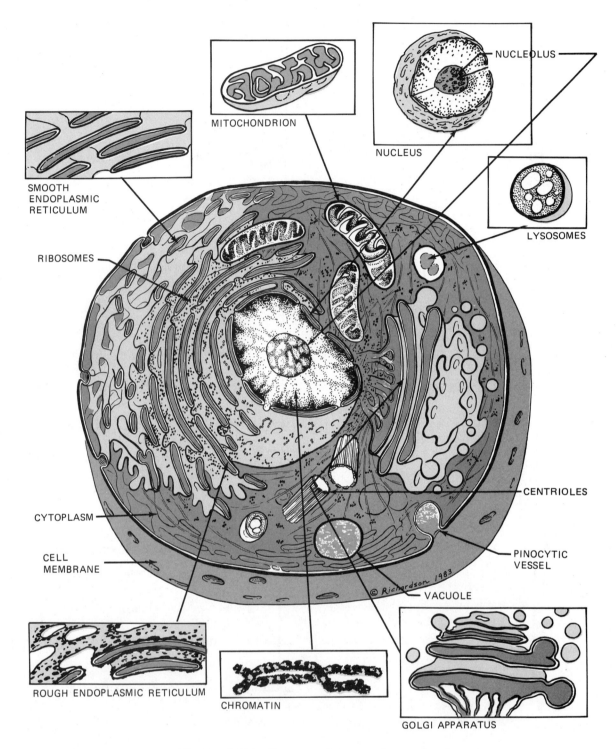

SMOOTH
ENDOPLASMIC
RETICULUM

MITOCHONDRION

NUCLEOLUS

NUCLEUS

LYSOSOMES

RIBOSOMES

CENTRIOLES

CYTOPLASM

PINOCYTIC
VESSEL

CELL
MEMBRANE

© Richardson 1983

VACUOLE

ROUGH ENDOPLASMIC RETICULUM

CHROMATIN

GOLGI APPARATUS

Figure 1–5   Structure of a typical animal cell

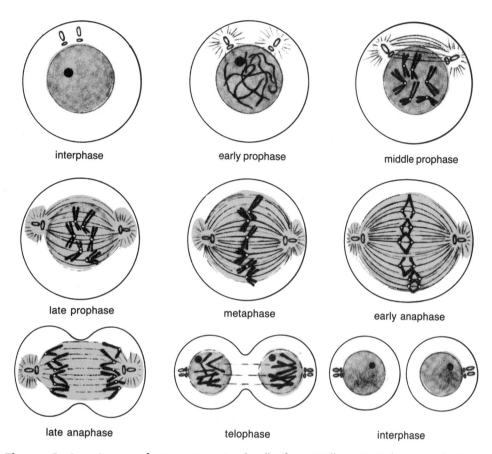

interphase   early prophase   middle prophase

late prophase   metaphase   early anaphase

late anaphase   telophase   interphase

Figure 1–6   Stages of mitosis in animal cells (from William D. Schraer and Herbert J. Stoltze, *Biology: The Study of Life*, 2nd ed. Copyright © 1987 by Allyn and Bacon, Inc.).

When the cell is ready to divide, the DNA and protein form short, rod-like structures called chromosomes. **Mitosis (meys-TOH-sis)** is the division process of cells, during which the nuclear material is distributed to each of the two new nuclei. The cytoplasm then divides into two, approximately equal, parts through the formation of a new membrane between the two nuclei. Mitosis is essentially an orderly series of steps by which the DNA in the nucleus of a cell is precisely and equally distributed to two "offspring" nuclei. (See Figure 1–6.)

Movement of Materials Across Cell Membranes

As previously mentioned, the cell membrane also controls the passage of substances into and out of the cell. This is important because the cell must acquire materials from its surroundings, after which it either secretes synthesized substances or excretes wastes. The physical processes involved in the passage of materials through the cell membrane are diffusion, osmosis, filtration, active transport, phagocytosis, and pinocytosis.

Diffusion   Diffusion is a physical, passive (requiring no energy in order to function)

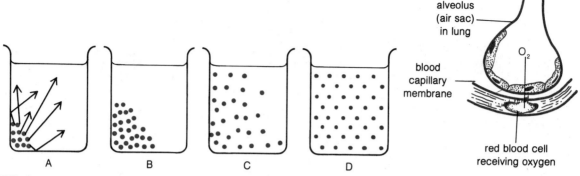

Diffusion:

(A) A small lump of sugar is placed into a beaker of water, its molecules dissolve and begin to diffuse outward. (B&C) The sugar molecules continue to diffuse through the water from an area of greater concentration to an area of lesser concentration. (D) Over a long period of time, the sugar molecules are evenly distributed throughout the water, reaching a state of equilibrium.

Example of diffusion in the human body: Oxygen diffuses from an alveolus in a lung where it is in greater concentration, across the blood capillary membrane, into a red blood cell where it is in lesser concentration.

Figure 1-7   The process of diffusion

process whereby molecules of gases, liquids, or solid particles disperse themselves evenly through a medium.

> **NOTE:** When solid particles are dissolved within a fluid, they are known as solutes.

Diffusion occurs due to the heat energy of molecules, and in all cases, the movement of molecules increases with increases in temperature. Diffusion plays a vital role in the ability of molecules to enter and leave a cell. For example, oxygen diffuses from the bloodstream, where it exists in greater concentration relative to oxygen in the cells. From the bloodstream, the oxygen enters the fluid surrounding a cell and then the cell itself, where it is much less concentrated. In this manner, the flow of blood through the lungs and bloodstream provides a continuous supply of oxygen to the cells. Once oxygen has entered a cell, it is used in metabolic activities. (See Figure 1–7.)

Osmosis   Osmosis is the diffusion of water or any other solvent molecule through a selective permeable membrane, such as a cell membrane. A selective permeable membrane is any membrane through which only certain solutes can diffuse. Osmotic pressure is the pressure developed when two solutions of different concentrations of the solute are separated by a membrane that is permeable only to the solvent. The osmotic pressure of a solution is dependent on the number of molecules of solute dissolved in a solution. The higher the osmotic pressure (osmolality) of a solution, the greater the number of molecules in that solution. (See Figure 1–8.)

Filtration   Filtration is the movement of solutes and water across a semipermeable membrane that results from some mechanical force such as blood pressure or gravity. Filtration allows for the separation of large and small molecules, as in the case of the

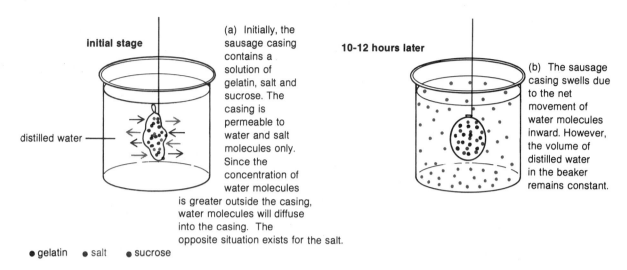

initial stage

distilled water —

(a) Initially, the sausage casing contains a solution of gelatin, salt and sucrose. The casing is permeable to water and salt molecules only. Since the concentration of water molecules is greater outside the casing, water molecules will diffuse into the casing. The opposite situation exists for the salt.

10-12 hours later

(b) The sausage casing swells due to the net movement of water molecules inward. However, the volume of distilled water in the beaker remains constant.

• gelatin • salt • sucrose

Figure 1-8   Osmosis, the diffusion of water through a selectively permeable membrane, is illustrated here. (A sausage casing is an example of a selectively permeable membrane.)

kidneys, where larger protein molecules are allowed to remain, while smaller molecules are excreted as waste.

Active Transport During active transport, the molecules move across the cell membrane via a carrier molecule which picks up a molecule on the outside of the cell membrane and then carries it back within the cell membrane. The molecule is then released at the inner surface of the membrane from where it enters the cytoplasm. The carrier acquires energy from the inner surface of the cell membrane, exits the membrane, and then begins the process again.

Phagocytosis (fay-goh-seye-TOH-sis) Phagocytosis is the process of the ingestion of foreign or other particles by certain cells. The material is completely enclosed within a vacuole, and digestive enzymes are produced from the cytoplasm to destroy the entrapped substance. **Pinocytosis (pin-oh-seye-TOH-sis)** is a similar process. However, the engulfed molecules are in a solution and, when they are destroyed, the cell ingests the nutrient for its own use.

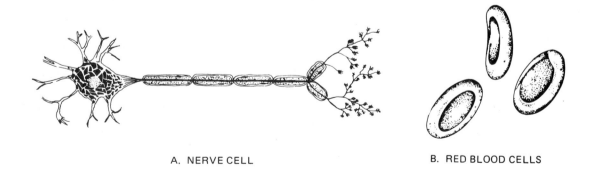

A. NERVE CELL

B. RED BLOOD CELLS

Figure 1-9   Specialized cells

Specialization

Most cells have the characteristics shown in Figure 1–5. However, some of the more specialized types of cells, such as nerve cells or red blood cells, may have a totally different structure. See Figure 1–9 for comparison.

Table 1–5   Different Kinds of Human Tissue

TYPE OF TISSUE	FUNCTION	CHARACTERISTICS AND LOCATION	MORPHOLOGY
I. EPITHELIAL	Cells form a continuous layer covering internal and external body surfaces, provide protection, produce secretions (digestive juices, hormones, perspiration) and regulate the passage of materials across themselves. A. **Covering and lining tissue** These cells can be stratified (layered), ciliated or keratinized.	1. **Squamous epithelial cells** These are flat, irregularly-shaped cells. They line the heart, blood and lymphatic vessels, body cavities, and alveoli (air sacs) of lungs. The outer layer of the skin is composed of stratified and keratinized squamous epithelial cells. The stratified squamous epithelial cells on the outer skin layer protect the body against microbial invasion.	I-A-1
		2. **Cuboidal epithelial cells** These are the cube-shaped cells that line the kidney tubules, and which cover the ovaries and secretory parts of certain glands.	I-A-2
		3. **Columnar epithelial cells** Elongated, with the nucleus generally near the bottom and often ciliated on the outer surface. They line the ducts, digestive tract (especially the intestinal and stomach lining), parts of the respiratory tract, and glands.	I-A-3

© Richardson 1983

Table 1-5   Different Kinds of Human Tissue (continued)

TYPE OF TISSUE	FUNCTION	CHARACTERISTICS AND LOCATION	MORPHOLOGY
I. EPITHELIAL (continued)	**B. Glandular or secretory tissue** These cells are specialized to secrete materials like digestive juices, hormones, milk, perspiration and wax. They are columnar or cuboidal shaped.	**Endocrine gland cells** These cells form ductless glands which secrete their substances (hormones) directly into the bloodstream. For instance, the thyroid gland secretes thyroxin, while adrenal glands secrete adrenalin. Exocrine glands secrete their substnaces into ducts. The mammary glands, sweat glands, and salivary glands are examples.	duct (where secretions leave) secretory cells exocrine (duct) gland cell e.g. sweat and mammary glands **I-B**
II. CONNECTIVE	Cells whose intercellular secretions (matrix) support and connect the many organs and tissues of the body.	Connective tissue is found almost everywhere within the body: bones, cartilage, mucous membranes, muscles, nerves, skin, and all internal organs.	cytoplasm collagen fibers nucleus vacuole (for fat storage)
	A. Adipose tissue Stores lipid (fat); acts as filler tissue; cushions, supports, and insulates the body.	A type of loose, connective tissue composed of sac-like adipose cells; they are specialized for the storage of fat. Adipose cells are found throughout the body: in the subcutaneous skin layer, around the kidneys, within padding around joints and in the marrow of long bones.	© Richardson 1983 **II-A**
	B. Areolar (loose) connective Surrounds various organs, supports both nerve cells and blood vessels which transport nutrient materials (to cells) and wastes (away from) cells. Areolar tissue also (temporarily) stores glucose, salts and water.	It is composed of a large, semifluid matrix, with many different types of cells and fibers embedded in it. These include fibroblasts (fibrocytes), plasma cells, macrophages, mast cells and various white blood cells. The fibers are bundles of a strong, flexible white fibrous protein called *collagen*, and elastic single fibers of *elastin*. It is found in the epidermis of the skin and in the subcutaneous layer with adipose (fat) cells.	matrix reticular fibers mast cell collagen fibers plasma cell elastic fiber fibroblast cell macrophage cell **II-B**

Table 1-5   Different Kinds of Human Tissue (continued)

TYPE OF TISSUE	FUNCTION	CHARACTERISTICS AND LOCATION	MORPHOLOGY
II. CONNECTIVE (continued)	**C. Dense fibrous** This tissue forms ligaments, tendons and aponeuroses. *Ligaments* are strong, flexible bands (or cords) which hold bones firmly together at the joints. *Tendons* are white, glistening bands attaching skeletal muscles to the bones. *Aponeuroses* are flat, wide bands of tissue holding one muscle to another or to the periosteum (bone covering). *Fasciae* are fibrous connective tissue sheets that wrap around muscle bundles to hold them in place.	Dense fibrous tissue is also called white fibrous tissue, since it is made from closely packed white collagen fibers. Fibrous tissue is flexible, but not elastic. It is found in aponeuroses, fasciae, ligaments and tendons.	closely packed collagen fibers fibroblast cell **II-C**
	D. Supportive **1. Bone (osseous) tissue —** Comprises the skeleton of the body, which supports and protects underlying soft tissue parts and organs, and also serves as attachments for skeletal muscles.	Connective tissue whose intercellular matrix is *calcified* by the deposition of mineral salts (like calcium carbonate and calcium phosphate). Calcification of bone imparts great strength. The entire skeleton is composed of bone tissue.	bone cell cytoplasm bone lacunae nucleus **II-D-1**
	2. Cartilage — Provides firm but flexible support for the embryonic skeleton and part of the adult skeleton. **a. Hyaline —** appears as a bluish white, glossy mass.	Hyaline cartilage is found upon articular bone surfaces, and also at the nose tip, bronchi and bronchial tubes. Ribs are joined to the *sternum* (breastbone) by the *costal cartilage.* It is also found in the larynx and the rings in the trachea.	matrix cells (chondrocytes) lacuna (space enclosing cells) **II-D-2a**
	b. Fibrocartilage — a strong, flexible, supportive substance; found between bones and wherever great strength (and a degree of rigidity) is needed.	Fibrocartilage is located within *intervertebral discs* and *pubic symphysis* between the *pubic bones.*	dense white fibers chondrocytes **II-D-2b**

© Richardson 1983

Table 1-5   Different Kinds of Human Tissue (continued)

TYPE OF TISSUE	FUNCTION	CHARACTERISTICS AND LOCATION	MORPHOLOGY
II. CONNECTIVE (continued)	**D. Supportive (continued)** **c. Elastic cartilage —** the intercellular matrix is embedded with a network of elastic fibers.	Elastic cartilage is located inside the auditory ear tube, external ear, epiglottis, and larynx.	*elastic fibers* *chondrocyte* *nucleus* © *Richardson 1983* **II-D-2c**
	E. Vascular (liquid blood tissue) **1. Blood —** Transports nutrient and oxygen molecules to cells, and metabolic wastes away from cells (can be considered as a liquid tissue). Contains cells that function in the body's defense and in blood clotting.	Blood is composed of two major parts: a liquid called plasma, and a solid cellular portion known as blood cells (or corpuscles). The plasma suspends corpuscles, of which there are two major types: *red* blood cells (erythrocytes) and *white* blood cells (leucocytes). A third cellular component (really a cell fragment) is called platelets (thrombocytes). Blood circulates within the blood vessels (arteries, veins and capillaries) and through the heart.	biconcave on both sides front view side view similar to a neutrophil but cytoplasmic granules are larger and stain with an acid dye like eosin granular leukocytes polymorphic nucleus polymorphic (lobulated) nucleus cytoplasmic granules stain with a basic dye cytoplasmic granules stain with a neutral dye basophil neutrophil eosinophil agranular leukocytes no cytoplasmic granules lymphocyte monocyte **II-E-1**
	2. Lymph — Transports tissue fluid, proteins, fats and other materials from the tissues to the circulatory system. This occurs through a series of tubes called the lymphatic vessels.	Lymph is a fluid made up of water, glucose, protein, fats and salt. The cellular components are lymphocytes and granulocytes. They flow in tubes called lymphatic vessels, which closely parallel the veins and bathe the tissue spaces between cells.	red blood cells white blood cell lymph cells © *Richardson 1983* lymph capillary **II-E-2**

Table 1–5   Different Kinds of Human Tissue (continued)

TYPE OF TISSUE	FUNCTION	CHARACTERISTICS AND LOCATION	MORPHOLOGY
III. **MUSCLE**	A. **Cardiac** These cells help the heart contract in order to pump blood through and out of the heart.	Cardiac muscle is a striated (having a cross-banding pattern), involuntary (not under conscious control) muscle. It makes up the walls of the heart.	III-A
	B. **Skeletal (striated voluntary)** These muscles are attached to the movable parts of the skeleton. They are capable of rapid, powerful contractions and long states of partially sustained contractions, allowing for voluntary movement.	Skeletal muscle is: *striated* (having transverse bands that run down the length of muscle fiber); *voluntary,* because the muscle is under conscious control; and *skeletal,* since these muscles are attached to the skeleton (bones, tendons and other muscles).	III-B
	C. **Smooth (nonstriated involuntary)** These provide for involuntary movement. Examples include the movement of materials along the digestive tract, controlling the diameter of blood vessels and the pupil of the eyes.	Smooth muscle is *nonstriated* because it lacks the striations (bands) of skeletal muscles; its movement is *involuntary.* It makes up the walls of the digestive, genitourinary, respiratory tracts, blood vessels and lymphatic vessels.	III-C
IV. **NERVE**	**Neuronal** Cells have the ability to react to stimuli. *Irritability —* ability of nerve tissue to respond to environmental changes. *Conductivity —* ability to carry a nerve impulse (message).	Nerve tissue is composed of neurons (nerve cells). Neurons have branches through which various parts of the body are connected and their activities coordinated. They are found in the brain, spinal cord, and nerves.	IV

© Richardson 1983

Tissues

Multicellular organisms are composed of many different types of cells that perform special functions. When cells are grouped according to their similarity in shape, size, and function they are called **tissues**. Some tissues are comprised of both living cells and nonliving substances that the cells build up around themselves. One such example is the supporting tissue near bones and cartilage.

The four main types of tissue—**epithelial (ep-ih-THEE-lee-al), connective, muscle**, and **nervous**—are depicted in Table 1–5, which provides the function, characteristics, and structural design of the four tissue types.

Table 1–6   The Ten Body Systems

SYSTEM	SYSTEM FUNCTIONS	ORGANS
Skeletal	Gives shape to body; protects delicate parts of body; provides space for attaching muscles; is instrumental in forming blood; stores minerals.	Skull, Spinal Column, Ribs and Sternum, Shoulder Girdle, Upper and Lower Extremities, Pelvic Girdle.
Muscular	Determines posture; produces body heat; provides for movement.	Voluntary Muscles (Skeletal) Involuntary Muscles Cardiac Muscle
Digestive	Prepares food for absorption and use by body cells through modification of chemical and physical states.	Mouth (salivary glands, teeth, tongue), Pharynx, Esophagus, Stomach, Intestines, Liver, Gallbladder, Pancreas.
Respiratory	Acquires oxygen; rids body of carbon dioxide.	Nose, Pharynx, Larynx, Trachea, Bronchi, Lungs.
Circulatory	Carries oxygen and nourishment to cells of body; carries waste from cells; body defense.	Heart, Arteries, Veins, Capillaries, Lymphatic Vessels, Lymph Nodes, Spleen.
Excretory	Removes waste products of metabolism from body.	Skin, Lungs, Kidneys, Bladder, Ureters, Urethra.
Nervous	Communicates; controls body activity, coordinates body activity.	Brain, nerves, Spinal Cord, Ganglia.
Endocrine	Manufactures hormones to regulate organ activity.	Glands (ductless): Pituitary, Thyroid, Parathyroid, Pancreas, Adrenal, Gonads (ovaries, testes)
Reproductive	Reproduces human beings.	*Male* — Testes, Scrotum, Epididymis, Vas deferens, Seminal vesicles, Ejaculatory duct, Prostate gland, Cowper's gland, Penis, Urethra *Female* — Ovaries, Fallopian tubes, Uterus, Vagina, Bartholin glands, External genitals (vulva), Breasts (mammary glands)
Integumentary	Helps regulate body temperature, establishes a barrier between the body and the environment; eliminates waste; synthesizes Vitamin D; contains receptors for temperature, pressure, and pain.	Epidermis, dermis, sweat glands, oil glands.

Organs and Systems

An organ is a structure comprised of several tissues grouped together to perform a single function. The organs of the body do not function separately, but instead coordinate their activities to form a complete, functional organism. Thus, a group of organs that act together to perform a specific and related function is known as an **organ system**.

The systems of the body are the skeletal, muscular, digestive, respiratory, circulatory, reproductive, excretory, endocrine, nervous, and integumentary systems. The functions and organs of each system can be studied by reviewing Table 1–6.

Tissue Repair

The repair of damaged tissues occurs continually, with some tissues undergoing repair more often then others. This is especially true of the skin which, during the course of daily living, is subjected to a lot of "wear and tear." Some tissues, such as surface epithelium, connective tissue, and liver cells, repair themselves quickly. Others, such as bone tissue, repair themselves slowly or minimally, as in the case of muscle tissue. Neurons (nerves) that are destroyed by infection or injury do not repair themselves or grow back. (See Table 1–7.)

There are two types of epithelial tissue repair—primary repair and secondary repair. Primary repair may consist of the normal new cell growth being pushed to the

Table 1–7   Vitamins Favorable to Tissue Repair

VITAMIN	FUNCTION
Vitamin A	Repairs epithelial tissue, especially the epithelial cells lining the respiratory tract.
Vitamin B (Thiamine, nicotinic acid, and riboflavin)	Helps to promote the general well-being of the individual. Specifically helps to promote appetite, metabolism, vigor, and pain relief in some cases.
Vitamin C	Helps in the normal production of and maintenance of collagen fibers and other connective tissue substances.
Vitamin D	Needed for the normal absorption of calcium from the intestine; possibly helps in the repair of bone fractures.
Vitamin K	Helps in the process of blood coagulation.
Vitamin E	Helps healing of tissues by acting as an antioxidant protector. It prevents important molecules and structures in the cell from reacting with oxygen. (When delicate components of living protoplasm are attacked by oxygen, they are literally "burnt.")

surface to repair the injury if the wound is clean. Deeper tissue damage may result in the need for sutures to bring the wound together so that the healing process can occur with minimal scarring.

Secondary repair concerns deeper, more serious wounds such as burns or mastectomies. In these cases, the individual must be kept immobile and in alignment while massive tissue repair is taking place.

The beauty care professional will more often than not be concerned with minor epithelial tissue injuries such as minor burns, cuts, and scrapes.

Burns There are three degrees of burns: first-degree, which is indicated by redness; second-degree, which includes redness, blisters, and swelling; and third-degree, when all layers of the skin are destroyed. Second- and third-degree burns require immediate medical attention.

The professional may find the following recommendations helpful in treatment of burns occurring in the workplace.

- Immediately put the burned area in cold water or apply a cold-water compress to the burn to reduce pain and swelling.
- Cover to minimize the risk of bacterial infection.
- Do not apply ointments or butter; do not break blisters.
- Protect the burn from exposure to the sun.

Integumentary System

The skin is a tough, pliable, and multifunctional covering for the underlying deeper tissues and provides protection from dehydration, injury, and invasion by germs. The skin also helps in the regulation of body temperature by either controlling the amount of heat loss or through the evaporation of perspiration to help rid the body of excess heat. Although only in minimal amounts, waste is also eliminated through the skin.

Blood and lymph supply nourishment to the skin, with one-half to two-thirds of the total blood supply being distributed to the skin. As the blood and lymph circulate through the skin, they contribute essential materials for its growth, nourishment, and repair.

The skin is sensitive to changes in its surrounding environment, which include changes in temperature—heat or cold, pain, pressure, and touch sensations.

Within the structure of the skin are tissues for the temporary storage of fat, glucose, water, and salts, subtances that are mostly later absorbed by the blood and transported to other areas of the body. Additionally, the skin is designed to act as a sunscreen for the harmful ultraviolet radiation contained in sunlight. The skin can also absorb certain drugs and chemical substances that can prove harmful, as in the case of insecticides, gasoline, or lead salts.

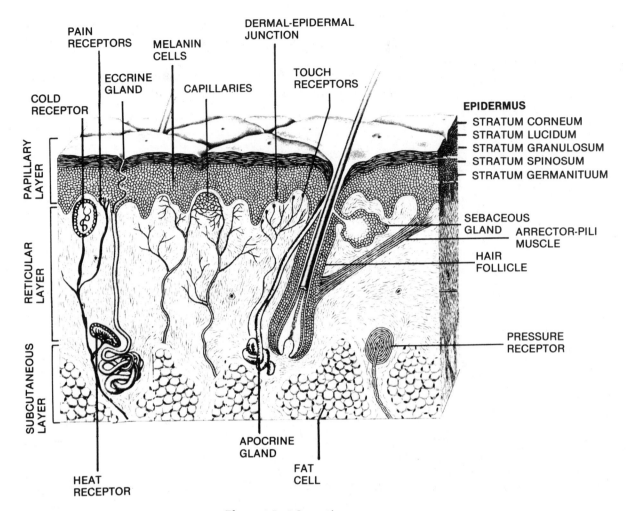

Figure 1-10   Skin structure

Structure of the Skin

The two basic layers of the skin are the epidermis, or cuticle, and the dermis corium, or true skin. (See Figure 1–10.)

Epidermis The epidermis forms the outer, protective covering of the skin, and although it does not contain blood vessels, it does have many small nerve endings. The epidermis consists of the stratum corneum, stratum lucidum, stratum granulosum, and stratum germinativum.

The **stratum corneum (STRAT-um kor-NEE-um)** forms the body's first line of defense against the invasion of bacteria, due to its slightly acidic properties, which can destroy many types of organisms on contact. Where cytoplasm would occur in other cells, in the cells that make up the stratum corneum, it is replaced by a nonliving protein substance called **keratin (KER-ah-tin)**, which acts as a waterproof covering. The cells of the stratum corneum are scale-like in appearance and tend to flake off from the constant friction of wearing clothing, washing, and similar activities. As these cells are shed, they are replaced by new cells from the underlying stratum germinativum.

> **NOTE:** The soft keratin found in the skin contains about 2 percent sulphur, 50 to 75 percent moisture, and a small percentage of fats.

The **stratum lucidum,** or clear layer, consists of small, transparent cells through which light can pass.

The **stratum granulosum** consists of cells that look like granules, are almost dead, and have undergone a change into a horny substance.

The **stratum germinativum** is an extremely important epidermal layer, as the replacement of cells in the epidermis depends on the division and growth of cells in this layer. These cells are then pushed up toward the stratum corneum, eventually becoming keratinized during the latter part of the process.

Found within the germinativum cells are **melanocytes (meh-LAN-oh-seyt)**, which contain a skin pigment known as **melanin (MEL-ah-nin)**. Melanin can be black, brown, or contain a yellowish cast, depending on the person's racial origin. An absence of melanin pigments (other than hemoglobin) results in albinism.

> **NOTE:** Melanin in the skin acts as a filter by darkening upon exposure. The phenomenon of tanning is simply the protective response of the skin to exposure to ultraviolet light.

The lower edge of the stratum germinativum is structured in ridges known as the **papillae (pah-PIL-ee)** of the skin. The papillae are most noticeable in the skin of the fingers, palms, and soles of the feet, where they actually raise the skin into permanent ridges. These ridges, which are referred to as friction ridges, provide maximum resistance against slippage when holding objects. Additionally, they provide individual and characteristic fingerprint patterns, which can be used for identification purposes.

Dermis The **dermis,** or corium (true skin), is the thicker, inner layer of the skin that contains matted masses of connective tissue; strong, fibrous tissue bands; elastic fibers (through which pass numerous blood vessels); lymphatics; nerve endings; muscles; hair follicles; oil and sweat glands; and fat cells.

There are also many different nerve receptors in the dermal layer, which include hot and cold sensory nerves as well as touch, pressure, and pain receptors. Pain receptors are located under the epidermis and around the hair follicles, being especially numerous on the lower arm, breast, and forehead. The dermis consists of two layers: the papillary and the reticular.

The **papillary** layer lies directly beneath the epidermis and contains cone-shaped projections of elastic tissue (papillae) that point upward into the epidermis. Some of the papillae contain looped capillaries, while others contain nerve fiber endings. This layer also contains some melanin skin pigment.

The **reticular** layer is thicker and more densely packed with fibers than the papillary layer. These fiber bundles are oriented horizontally, rather than vertically as in the papillary layer, and contain the following structures: fat cells, blood vessels, lymph vessels, oil glands, sweat glands, hair follicles, and arrector pili muscles.

Below the dermis is a layer of fatty tissue known as **subcutaneous (sub-kyoo-TAY-**

nee-us) tissue which provides contour to the body, contains fats for energy, and acts as a protective cushion for the outer skin. The circulation to this layer is maintained by a network of arteries and lymphatics.

The professional working with skin on a regular basis should be aware that **collagen (KAWL-ah-jen)** *makes up about 70 percent of the dermis. Within the dermis, it forms a network of interwoven fibers that give the skin structural support for cells and blood vessels, allows for stretching and contraction of the skin, and aids in the healing of wounds. The space between the collagen fibers contains a protein called* **elastin** *that provides the skin with elasticity. Collagen is a binder of water and therefore helps reduce the amount of moisture lost by the skin; however, moisture is essential to keeping the collagen network supple. The balance and maintenance of moisture is one of the most influential aspects of beautiful skin. It is the condition of the skin's collagen, and not the facial muscles, that influences the formation of lines and wrinkles. With age, the collagen network begins to weaken, losing moisture and resiliency, which causes the skin to lose its tone and suppleness.*

Reticulin is another fibrous protein that works with collagen and elastin to give the dermis its elasticity, resilience, and strength. Although the exact function of reticulin is not fully understood, it is thought to help the collagen fibrils to form properly.

Appendages of the Skin

The **appendages of the skin** are the hair, nails, sweat glands, and sebaceous (oil) glands and their ducts.

Hair   Hair is distributed over most of the surfaces of the body. For an in-depth study of the structure and growth of hair, please refer to Chapter 2.

The Nails   The **nails** (onyz, onych) are hard structures of keratinized plates (the hardest form of keratin) that cover the dorsal surfaces of the last phalanges (bones) of the fingers and toes. A nail is formed in the nail bed, or **matrix**, where the cells first appear as elongated cells until they are fused together to form the keratinized plates, which serve to protect the tips of the fingers and toes. This plate does not contain nerves or blood vessels. Healthy nails are smooth, shiny, and translucent pink. Systemic problems in the body can show in the nails as disorders or poor nail growth. Nails replace themselves every five to six months and tend to grow faster in the summer.

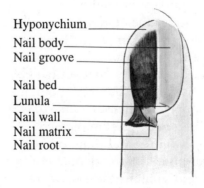

Hyponychium
Nail body
Nail groove

Nail bed
Lunula
Nail wall
Nail matrix
Nail root

Figure 1–11   Diagram of a nail

The entire nail structure consists of parts of the actual nail and structures of skin beneath and surrounding the nail. (See Figure 1–11.)

The actual nails consists of the nail body, nail root, and free edge. The **nail body** or **plate** is the main part of nail and is attached to the skin at the tip of the finger. Although the nail appears to be one piece, it is actually constructed of layers.

The **nail root** is the point where the nail growth begins. It is embedded underneath the skin at the base of the nail.

The **free edge** is the end of the nail that extends beyond the fingertip.

The structures beneath the nail include the nail bed, matrix, and lunula. The **nail bed** is the portion of skin beneath the nail body on which the nail plates rests. The nail bed is supplied with blood vessels that provide the nourishment necessary for nail growth. The nail bed also contains nerves.

The **matrix (MAY-triks)** contains nerves together with lymph and blood vessels which produce nail cells and control the rate of growth of the nail. It is located under the nail root. The matrix is a very sensitive part of the nail and if injured, it will produce nails with irregular growth and disorders. Be careful not to apply excessive pressure to this area during a manicure.

The **lunule (LOO-nyool)** is the light-colored half-moon shape at the base of the nail. This is the point where the matrix connects with the nail bed.

The skin surrounding the nail includes the cuticle, nail fold, nail grooves, nail wall, eponychium, perionychium, and hyponychium.

The **cuticle (KYOO-ti-kel)** is the overlapping skin around the nail. A normal cuticle should be loose and pliable.

The **nail fold** or **mantle (MAN-tel)** is the deep fold of skin at the base of the nail where the nail root is imbedded.

The **nail grooves** are slits or tracks in the nail bed at the sides of the nail on which the nail grows.

The **nail wall** is the skin on the sides of the nail above the grooves.

The **eponychium (ep-o-NIK-ee-um)** is the thin line of skin at the base of the nail that extends from the nail wall to the nail plate.

The **perionychium (per-ee-o-NIK-ee-um)** is the part of the skin bordering the root and the sides of the nail.

The **hyponychium (heye-poh-NIK-ee-um)** is the part of the skin under the free edge of the nail.

> *The professional who performs manicures or pedicures should not perform massage if the client has high blood pressure or a heart condition or has had a stroke. Massage increases circulation and may be harmful to such a client. Also avoid vigorous massage if the client has arthritis.*

Occasionally, a nail is lost due to disease or injury; however, as long as the nail bed remains intact, a new nail will form.

Sweat Glands   There are two types of **sweat** or **sudoriferous (soo-doh-RIF-er-us) glands**—apocrine and eccrine—which are separate structures and have different functions.

Apocrine glands are the larger of the two types. They empty into the canal of the

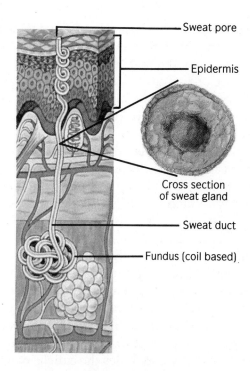

Sweat pore

Epidermis

Cross section
of sweat gland

Sweat duct

Fundus (coil based)

Figure 1-12   Sweat gland

follicle at a point above the sebaceous duct in the armpit, pubic areas, and outside ear canals. Apocrine secretion is stimulated only by emotional stress.

Eccrine sweat glands are most numerous on the palms, soles of the feet, and the head. The eccrine ducts open directly onto the surface of the skin, where they secrete large amounts of diluted salt water when stimulated by heat or emotional stress.

Excretion is a minor function of the skin through which certain wastes, dissolved in perspiration, are removed. Perspiration consists of 99 percent water with only trace amounts of salt and organic materials (waste products).

In structure, sweat glands are tubular with a coiled base and a tubelike duct, which extends to form a pore in the skin. Sweat glands are under the control and influence of the nervous system, which can be activated by such factors as heat, pain, fever, and nervousness or anxiety, resulting in perspiration being excreted through the pores. When exercise or exertion result in profuse sweating and water loss, it is vital to replace the fluids as soon as possible. (See Figure 1–12.)

Sebaceous (seh-BAY-shus) Oil Glands   The sebaceous glands secrete a thick, oily substance known as **sebum (SEE-bum)**, which lubricates the skin, maintaining its softness and pliability.

The Skin and Its Relationship to Bacteria

Most of the skin surface is unfavorable for bacterial growth due to its dryness. However, in moist skin areas, such as around the hair follicle or sweat glands, where nutrients are present and moisture content high, skin bacteria can adhere and grow on the surfaces of dead cells that compose the outer epidermal layer. The types of microbes found are usually of the Staphylococcus, Corynebacterium, yeast, or fungi species.

> **NOTE:** Depending on the skin condition and number of microbes present, it takes seven to eight minutes of scrubbing to remove most temporary skin bacteria. More permanent, or resident, bacteria may not be so easily removed, as washing may actually draw out bacteria that were embedded in the hair follicles. To achieve optimum cleanliness, an antibacterial soap or solution should be used.

The professional should be aware that absorption by the skin is accomplished through the indentations of the hair follicles and the pores of the sweat glands. These pockets will allow the entry of certain drugs, chemicals, and solutions into the body, which may combat infection or moisturize the skin. Maintaining moisture in the skin may be a problem for some individuals. Deficiencies may be caused either by an inadequate diet, drying cleansing agents, or underactivity of sebum from the sebaceous glands. Sebum is important in maintaining moisture content because as it coats the skin surface, it helps slow down the evaporation of water.

Additionally, the skin is a breathing organ because it takes in oxygen and discharges carbon dioxide. The skin should never be entirely coated with any substance (such as paint) that interferes with this breathing process.

Fill in the Blank

1. Two types of anatomical study that the professional may practice when performing typical services are _____ and _____.

2. _____ is the study of the structure, function, and development of cells.

3. _____ is the study of tissues and organs of an entire body organism.

4. Angiology is the study of the _____ system.

5. Arthrology is the study of the _____.

6. Myology is the study of the _____ system.

7. Neurology is the study of the _____ system.

8. Five areas of study that relate to the performance of massage movements and treatments are the _____, _____, _____, _____, and _____.

9. Four major subcavities of the body are the _____, _____, _____, and _____ cavities.

10. The cranial and spinal cavities are located within the _____ cavity.

11. The thoracic and abdominopelvic cavities are found in the _____ cavity.

12. Three smaller cavities with which the professional may be concerned are the _____, _____, and _____ cavities.

13. Nerves and muscles in the orbital, nasal, and buccal cavities are highly influenced by _____, _____, _____, _____, and the _____.

14. Odors may cause _____ reactions when inhaled.

15. The 12 vital life functions are _____, _____, _____, _____, _____, _____, _____, _____, _____, _____, _____, and _____.

16. Living depends on the constant release of _____ derived from _____.

17. _____ are special cells grouped according to function, shape, size, and structure.

18. Tissues form units known as _____ .

19. Metabolism is the total process of the _____ within a cell.

20. Metabolism consists of two opposite processes, _____ and _____ .

21. _____ may be grouped together to perform a related function.

22. The functioning of the human body requires the combined activities of _____ , _____ , _____ , and _____ .

23. The three states, or phases, in which matter can exist are _____ , _____ , and _____ .

24. _____ are the basic building blocks of all matter.

25. Four elements that make up 97 percent of all living matter are _____ , _____ , _____ , and _____ .

26. _____ are formed when elements are combined together in specific proportions of weight.

27. _____ are the smallest units of a compound that still have the properties of the compound.

28. The two groups of compounds are _____ and _____ .

29. Inorganic compounds do not generally contain the element _____ .

30. _____ compounds always contain the element carbon.

31. Carbohydrates contain the elements _____ , _____ , and _____ .

32. _____ are single, or simple, sugars that cannot be broken down further.

33. _____ , _____ , and _____ are examples of monosaccharides.

34. Examples of double sugars include _____ , _____ , and _____ .

35. Polysaccharides are found in, or made by, _____ .

36. Three examples of polysaccharides are _____ , _____ , and _____ .

37. Lipids differ from carbohydrates in that they have _____ oxygen than hydrogen.

38. _____ are one of the most essential organic compounds found in all living organisms.

39. Proteins are composed of smaller molecular units called _____ .

40. There are _____ essential amino acids that the body cannot produce.

41. Enzymes are specialized protein molecules that help to control _____ occurring within the cell.

42. Two examples of nucleic acids are _____ and _____ .

43. An _____ is a substance that will ionize when dissolved in water.

44. A base, or alkali, ionizes into negatively charged _____ and positively charged ions of a metal.

45. When an acid and a base are combined, they form a _____.

46. The term pH means _____.

47. The pH scale is used to measure the _____ or _____ of a solution.

48. The pH scale ranges from _____ to _____.

49. A pH of 7 indicates that the solution has _____ amounts of hydrogen ions and hydroxide ions, resulting in a _____ pH level.

50. In living organisms, pH balance is maintained through a compound called a _____.

51. _____ and _____ are ingredient substances with which the professional should be familiar in order to recommend products.

52. The _____ is the basic unit of structure and function of all living things.

53. The _____ is the background for all the chemical reactions within a cell.

54. Two chemical reactions occurring within the cytoplasm are _____ and _____.

55. The most important organelle, or cell structure, within a cell is the _____.

56. Two vital functions of the nucleus are to control the _____ of the cell and to facilitate _____.

57. The division process of cells is known as _____.

58. The _____ controls the passage of substances into and out of the cell.

59. Diffusion occurs due to the _____ of molecules.

60. _____ is the diffusion of a solvent through a selective permeable membrane.

61. _____ is the movement of solutes and water across a semipermeable membrane via a mechanical force such as blood pressure or gravity.

62. Two specialized cells that maintain totally different structures than most cells are the _____ and the _____.

63. Enter the names of the structures after the proper numbered callouts, as listed below.

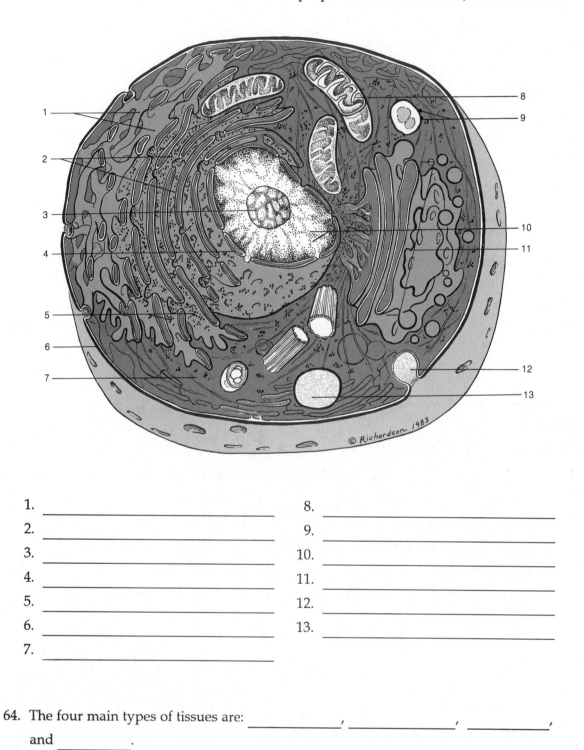

1. _____	8. _____
2. _____	9. _____
3. _____	10. _____
4. _____	11. _____
5. _____	12. _____
6. _____	13. _____
7. _____	

64. The four main types of tissues are: _____, _____, _____, and _____.

65. _____ tissue performs the following functions: covers internal and external body surfaces, provides protection, produces secretions, and regulates the passage of materials across themselves.

66. _____ tissue supports and connects organs and tissues of the body.

67. The three types of muscular tissue are _____ , _____ , and

    _____ .

68. An _____ is a structure comprised of several tissues grouped together to perform
    a single function.

69. When a group of organs act together to perform a specific and related function, it is
    known as an _____ .

70. The ten systems of the body are the _____ , _____ , _____ ,

    _____ , _____ , _____ , _____ , _____ ,

    _____ , and _____ .

71–80. Identify the following organs with the system to which each belongs:

71. _____   Voluntary skeletal muscles

72. _____   Mouth

73. _____   Heart

74. _____   Spinal column

75. _____   Lungs

76. _____   Spinal cord

77. _____   Kidneys

78. _____   Epidermis

79. _____   Glands

80. _____   Breasts

81. The two types of epithelial repair are _____ repair and _____ repair.

82. The professional will be concerned with epithelial tissue injuries such as

    _____ , _____ , and _____ .

83. When treating a minor burn, apply _____ to reduce swelling and pain.

84. The function of the skin is to provide protection from _____ , _____ ,

    and _____ .

85. The skin helps in the _____ of body temperature.

86. Small amounts of _____ are eliminated through the skin.

87. Tissues in the skin provide storage for _____ , _____ , _____ , and

    _____ .

88. The _____ acts as a sunscreen for harmful ultraviolet rays.

89. The skin can absorb _____ and _____ .

90. The two basic layers of the skin are the _____ and the _____ .

91. The epidermis consists of four layers, the _____ , _____ ,
    _____ , and _____ .

92. _____ in the stratum corneum acts as a waterproof covering.

93. The _____ consists of the reproductive layers of the epidermis.

94. Melanin is a skin pigment found in the _____ and the
    _____ layer of the skin.

95. Tanning is the protective response of the skin to _____ .

96. The dermis consists of two layers, the _____ and the _____ .

97. The _____ layer contains projections of elastic tissues called papillae, looped
    capillaries, nerve fiber endings, and some melanin.

98. The _____ layer contains fat cells, blood vessels, lymph vessels, oil glands,
    sweat glands, hair follicles, and arrector pili muscles.

99. A layer of fatty tissue lying below the dermis is known as _____ .

100. Collagen makes up about _____ percent of the dermis.

101. It is the condition of the skin's _____ that causes lines and wrinkles.

102. _____ is a protein that provides the skin with elasticity.

103. The appendages of the skin are the _____ , _____ , _____ , and
     _____ and their _____ .

104. Nails are hard structures of _____ plates.

105. A nail is formed in the nail bed, or _____ .

106. The two types of sweat glands are the _____ and the _____ .

107. _____ glands empty into the follicle canal.

108. _____ glands open directly onto the surface of the skin.

109. Apocrine secretion is stimulated only by _____ .

110. Eccrine secretion is stimulated by _____ or _____ .

111. Sweat glands are under the control and influence of the _____ system.

112. Sebaceous glands secrete _____ .

113. Sebum _____ the skin.

114. The types of _____ found on skin are usually of the Staphylococcus, Coryne-
     bacterium, yeast, or fungus varieties.

115. The average amount of scrubbing time it takes to remove temporary skin bacteria is
     _____ to _____ minutes.

2

Physiology and Histology of the Hair

A thorough understanding of the physiology and histology of the hair is of vital importance to professionals who perform hair services and treatments on a daily basis. This also includes services that may influence the ultimate nature of subsequent hair shafts, such as scalp treatments and massage.

Follicle Formation

The growth of hair is enabled by the development of small downgrowths into the dermis starting at approximately the beginning of the third month of fetal life. These downgrowths of the epidermis are called **follicles (FAWL-ih-kels)**. By the fifth or sixth month, the follicles have produced soft, downy hair called **lanugo (lah-NOO-goh)** or **primary hair**. Most of the lanugo hair is shed prior to birth except in the regions of the eyebrows, eyelids, and scalp.

Several months after birth, the body develops a second hair growth. Known as **vellus (VELL-us)**, this is the protective, fine hair that covers the body later in life. The original lanugo hair of the scalp, eyebrows, and eyelids also goes through a shedding and regrowth process, producing **secondary hair** which is more stiff and bristly than the lanugo hair.

Tertiary (TER-she-air-ee) or **terminal hair** is the long, soft hair found on the scalp, the beard and mustache of adult males, and the legs and underarms of all adults.

Each of the three main types of hair, lanugo, secondary, and terminal, has its own special features. The distinction is usually based on the length and texture of the hair. It does not appear that different types of follicles produce these hairs, but rather that they result from changes in the body and, subsequently, in the papilla. Most of these changes are due to genetic factors, age, hormones, and at times, hormonal imbalances in the body.

> **NOTE:** Some experts use the terms *lanugo* and *vellus* interchangeably. Others feel these is a distinction between the two and limit *lanugo* to the downy hairs covering the body of the fetus, especially when premature.

Listed below are the main features of each hair type.

Primary Hair

There are several distinctive features of primary hair. They are:

1. Lack of medulla.

2. Lack of pigment, which makes the hair difficult to see unless it is examined in a strong light at the proper angle.
3. Absence of arrector pili muscles, although sebaceous glands are present.
4. Short length: each hair is usually about a half inch (1.25 cm).

The function of primary hair is to aid in the evaporation of perspiration on the body.

Secondary Hair

Secondary hair is the stiff, short, bristly hair of the eyelashes and eyebrows. It can also be found inside the nose and ears, under the arms, and in the pubic area.

The follicles of these hairs usually lie at right angles to the surface of the skin, so that the hairs stand straight out away from the skin. They do not possess arrector pili muscles. The main features of secondary hairs are:

1. A probable increase in thickness and number with age, particularly in the eyebrows and edges of the ears of older males.
2. A curved shape in many cases.
3. A large medulla in many cases.
4. A hair-length range of between 1/2 inch and 3/4 inch (1.25 cm and 1.87 cm).
5. More sensitivity to the touch than scalp hairs, enabling them to act as protection for the eyes, ears, and nose.
6. They are not lost in the normal balding process.

The function of secondary hair is protection. The hair of the eyelashes is controlled by very sensitive reflex actions that help prevent foreign objects from entering the eye. The eyebrow hair serves to divert liquids from the eye. The hair of the nose and ears serves as protection against bacteria entering the body. Underarm (axillary) hair and pubic hair also fall into this category.

Tertiary Hair

Tertiary hair (also known as terminal hair) is the long, soft, thick hair found on the scalp. It can also be found on the beard and mustache of adult males, and on the legs, arms, and body of both males and females. These hairs grow in groups of two to five, especially on the scalp. In these groups, the hairs may be of different ages and lengths.

The follicles of these long, soft hairs lie at an angle to the skin, which accounts for the growth direction of the hair. Sometimes, several follicles merge together to form one opening on the skin surface. This results in multiple hairs or what appears to be several hairs coming from one follicle.

Tertiary hair is pigmented. It is only in the cases of albinism, aging, glandular disorders, and hereditary traits that tertiary hair is white or gray. This type of hair often possesses a natural wave.

Each hair has at least one sebaceous gland associated with the follicle. The function of the gland is to produce a natural oil (sebum). This oil forms a film on the outside of the hair shaft and the outer layer of the epidermis. Each hair has arrector pili muscles and so is able to demonstrate the characteristic "goose bumps."

Tertiary hair of the scalp will thin with age and in cases where the patient has excess amounts of the male hormone testosterone. Some experts believe that these people will eventually bald and that the tertiary hairs on other areas of the body will become longer, thicker, and more pigmented.

> *The ability to recognize the characteristics of the three basic hair types assists the professional in the diagnostic aspects of determining abnormal hair growth or placement, especially as related to female clients. In many cases, tertiary hair on the face of a female may appear following hormonal changes or imbalances, in places where previously, only lanugo hair was present. A correct analysis of the hair type will help to determine the type of treatment, its duration, and the probability of success.*

Structure of the Follicle

The hair follicle surrounds the hair root and is made up of external and internal root sheaths. The external root sheath is a downward continuation of the epidermis. At the bottom of the hair follicle, the external root sheath contains only the stratum basale, a single layer of columnar cells capable of continued cell division, and part of the stratum germinativum of the skin (or epidermis). The internal root sheath is formed from the cells of the matrix (a germinal layer at the base of the hair bulb) and takes the form of a cellular, tubular sheath that separates the hair from the external root sheath. The internal root sheath extends only partway up the follicle. (See Figure 2–1.)

The follicle does not dip directly downward at right angles to the skin, but rather is sloped at a slight angle. A small muscle, called the arrector pili muscle, is attached to one side of the follicle approximately one-third of the way down from the skin surface. This muscle contracts under stresses induced by fright, cold, or emotion and pulls the hairs into a vertical position, while the skin around the shaft forms slight elevations, resulting in "goose bumps." (See Figure 2–2.)

> *When performing electrology treatments, the angle of the hair growth must be considered in order to correctly determine the angle of the needle during insertion. If the hair possesses a natural wave, it will need to be cut short in order to judge the growth direction of the hair. When discussing follicle structure, it is also important to note that the arrector pili muscle is destroyed during the electrology process, with the result that "goose bumps" will no longer form in the treated area.*

The follicles are not scattered evenly on the scalp but rather are grouped together. These groups may contain two to five hairs each, although sometimes the mouths of two separate follicles come together. This makes it appear that two hairs are growing from the same follicle (compound hairs); however, each hair still has its own individual papilla at the bottom of each follicle.

NOTE: Some hair follicles produce hairs in abnormal situations, such as the disturbance of glands and hereditary disorders. Glands help regulate hormones. If the chemical balance of glands is disturbed or altered due to medications or a physiological condition, this can have an adverse effect on the system.

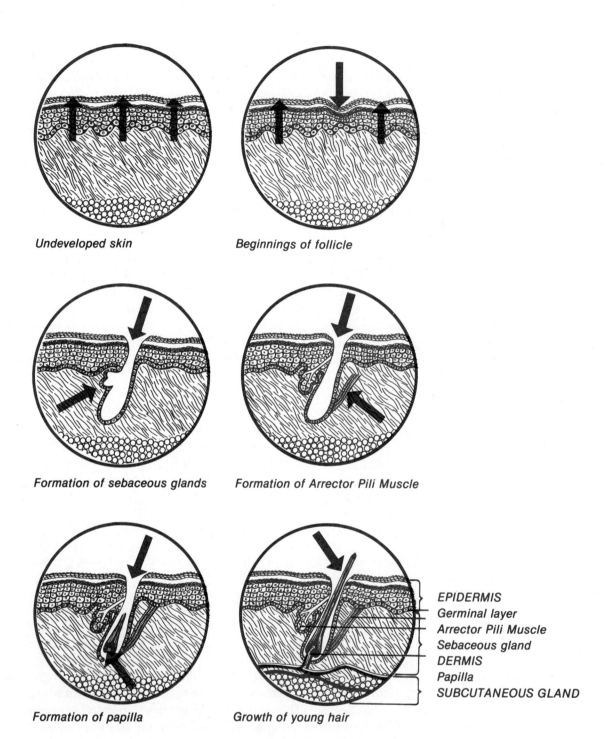

Undeveloped skin   Beginnings of follicle

Formation of sebaceous glands   Formation of Arrector Pili Muscle

Formation of papilla   Growth of young hair

EPIDERMIS
Germinal layer
Arrector Pili Muscle
Sebaceous gland
DERMIS
Papilla
SUBCUTANEOUS GLAND

Figure 2-1   Origin of the follicle and hair

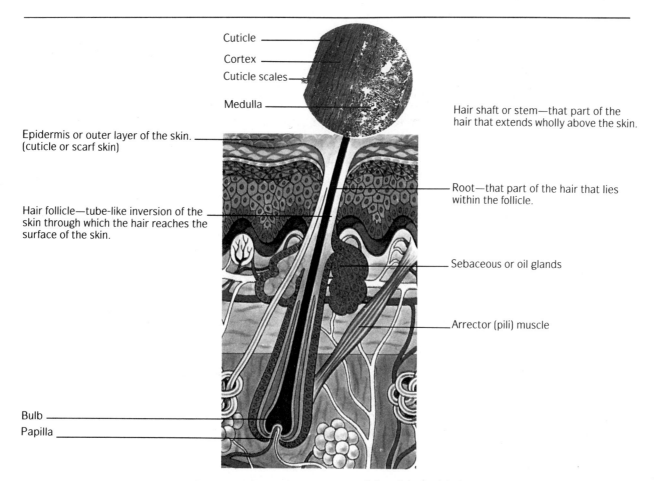

Cuticle

Cortex

Cuticle scales

Medulla

Hair shaft or stem—that part of the hair that extends wholly above the skin.

Epidermis or outer layer of the skin. (cuticle or scarf skin)

Root—that part of the hair that lies within the follicle.

Hair follicle—tube-like inversion of the skin through which the hair reaches the surface of the skin.

Sebaceous or oil glands

Arrector (pili) muscle

Bulb

Papilla

Figure 2-2   Cross section of the skin and hair

Further down the follicle structure is a network of nerves that are directly connected to the brain. If a live hair is plucked from the follicle, these nerves transmit a message of pain.

Hair Root

The hair root is the portion of the hair located within the follicle. Its structure includes the hair bulb and the papilla.

The hair bulb is a thickened, club-like structure forming the lower part of the hair root. Melanin, the pigment in hair, is produced by special cells of the hair bulb. As the hair grows upward, the pigment is carried into the cortex of the forming hair. Many experts feel that the lack of color in lanugo hair is due to the lack of a hair bulb. The lower part of the hair bulb is hollowed out to fit over and cover the hair papilla.

The papilla is a cone-shaped elevation of loose, connective tissue that is richly supplied with blood and nerves. It provides nourishment to the hair bulb and is responsible for hair growth and regeneration.

The other portion of the papilla comes in contact with the germinal matrix and transfers nutrients to the germinativa cells. The cells are able to change their food materials into keratin to form the hair. As long as the papilla functions, the hair will continue to grow.

> *Since hair will continue to grow as long as the papilla functions, it is important during electrolysis to destroy at least the bottom third of the follicle in order to ensure that the papilla will not create new cells, thus producing a new hair.*

NOTE: Everyone is born with a set number of hair follicles, and while new hair can grow from dormant hair follicles, new follicles are never formed.

Other Structures Connected with the Follicle

Sebaceous (or oil) glands consist of sac-like structures situated in the dermis that are connected to the hair follicle by the sebaceous duct. The ducts secrete an oily substance called sebum, which is a mixture of fats, cholesterol, proteins, and inorganic salts. Sebum gives luster and pliability to the hair and keeps the skin soft and flexible. Much of the activity of the sebaceous gland is controlled by the endocrine system, and gland overactivity (especially after puberty) can be an indication of glandular problems and may be the cause of excess hair.

NOTE: When sebaceous glands of the face become enlarged because of accumulated sebum, blackheads develop. The color of blackheads is due to the combination of melanin and oxidized oil, and is not necessarily dirt. Pimples and boils may result because sebum is nutritive to certain bacteria.

Sudoriferous (Sweat) Glands

The principal function of the sudoriferous gland is to help regulate body temperature, although it also helps to eliminate wastes from the body. Both functions are brought about by the production of perspiration or sweat in the glands. This is a mixture of water, salts, urea, uric acid, amino acids, ammonia, sugar, lactic acid, and ascorbic acid.

In contrast to the sebaceous glands, sudoriferous glands are most abundant in the skin of the palms and soles of the feet. Their density in these areas can be as high as 3,000 per square inch. Sudoriferous glands are also found in the armpits and the forehead. These glands consist of a coiled end embedded primarily in the dermis. A single duct projects upward through the dermis and epidermis, terminating in a pore at the surface of the skin. The base of a sudoriferous gland is surrounded by a network of small blood vessels. (See Figure 2–3.)

The Structure of the Hair

Hair consists of a special arrangement of hard keratin developed by the reproduction of cells from the germinal (matrix) layers of the skin in the hair follicle. As the cells move up the follicle, the amino acids ("the building blocks" of all protein) that they contain join together to create the three principal components of the hair fiber: the cuticle, the cortex, and the medulla.

The Cuticle

The **cuticle (KYOO-ti-kel)** is the outside layer of the hair shaft. It consists of hard, flattened scales that overlap one another with an average thickness of seven scales.

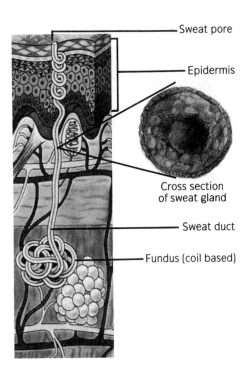

- Sweat pore
- Epidermis
- Cross section of sweat gland
- Sweat duct
- Fundus (coil based)

Figure 2-3   Sweat gland

This arrangement of overlapping scales, called **imbrications**, points upward and outward in the direction of hair growth and provides the hair with strength and flexibility. The imbrications also act as reservoirs for the sebum supply while functioning as protection for the more delicate cortex.

When performing hair services, the professional should be aware that the structure of the cuticle is the element of hair form that allows for the easy removal by brushing of undesirable material such as dirt, scalp cells, or flaking skin. The cuticle also acts as a base for the deposit of hair sprays, conditioners, fillers, temporary color, and other hair cosmetics. During a hair analysis prior to conditioning or chemical treatments, testing of the imbrications may be accomplished by sliding the thumb and index finger lengthwise on the hair strand from end to root for the purpose of checking porosity and texture. Loose, open scales will indicate greater porosity and the ability to absorb moisture, while tight, firm scales indicate a more "closed" cuticle, which offers more resistance to the penetration of products and chemicals. (See Figure 2–4.)

The Cortex

The physical structure of the **cortex** is a complicated formation of many millions of parallel fibers of hard keratin, referred to as polypeptide chains, that twist around one another in a rope fashion. The cortex is the most important layer of the hair, forming 75 percent to 90 percent of its bulk, or mass, and it is responsible for most of the "behavior" of human hair. This behavior includes such characteristics as the

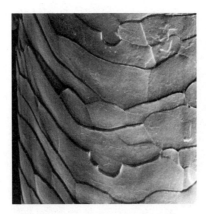

Figure 2–4   Magnified view of the hair cuticle, which is composed of keratin

amount of natural "body" of the hair; its ability to take a perm, color, or other chemical treatments; and its general health.

The physical properties of the hair that depend upon the cortex are:

1. strength,
2. elasticity,
3. pliability,
4. direction and manner of growth,
5. size or diameter,
6. texture and quality,
7. color, and
8. wave.

Strength. Because of the nature of the cortex, hair has great strength and elasticity. In fact, it is claimed that human hair is stronger than copper wire of the same diameter. A single strand of hair in good condition will support a weight of approximately five to seven ounces.

Elasticity. The coil structure of the fibers of the cortex also account for the hair's elasticity. The coils are interlocked by hydrogen and sulphur bonds, which allow it to be stretched and then ensure that it returns to its normal shape.

Pliability. The pliability of the hair will depend on a combination of all its physical properties with the possible exception of color. Strength, elasticity, direction of growth, diameter, texture, and natural wave all help determine how pliable or susceptible the hair will be to new formation or direction.

Direction and Manner of Growth. Although the direction in which hair grows is due to the angle or slant of the follicle, it should be remembered that the factor that most influences follicle design is genetic and hereditary in nature. Most professional stylists will agree that working with the hair growth rather than against it is the best approach to hairstyle design.

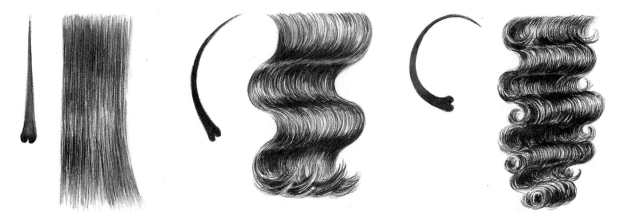

Figure 2-5   Straight hair, wavy hair, and curly hair

Diameter or Size. The mass of the hair is due to the amount of fibers in the cortex, which is determined by age, health, and hereditary traits.

Texture and Quality. The texture and quality of the hair will depend on genetic factors, general internal health, the amount of sebum and natural moisture in the hair, and its strength, diameter, elasticity, pliability, type (lanugo, secondary, or tertiary hair), and location on the body.

Color. The natural color of the hair is due to melanin granules that are produced at a specialized site on the hair bulb. These granules are released and are trapped in the forming cortex. Lanugo and vellus hairs do not have pigmentation, probably due to incomplete development of the hair root.

Wave. The natural curl pattern of the hair is due to the growth pattern of hair cells in the root. Experts state that genetic factors cause one side of the papilla to produce cells faster, causing uneven growth. The twisting of the fibers into coils (helices) results in a wave pattern. (See Figure 2–5.)

How the Cortex and the Cuticle Work Together

The cortex and the cuticle are the two main parts of the hair, consisting of different arrangements of hard keratin, with each layer performing separate and distinct functions. Although the structures and functions may differ, there exists an essential interdependence between the two which is illustrated in the following examples:

1. The cuticle is tough and will resist wear or friction but it has no strength.
2. The cortex has great strength but is not tough or able to resist wear or friction.
3. The cuticle protects the cortex but does not hold it together. The cortex holds together very well but is easily damaged.
4. The *cuticle allows waving and setting* to take place, but *only the cortex is able to be waved or set.*
5. The cuticle allows the hair to be stretched, but only the cortex is elastic.
6. The cortex requires a certain amount of moisture to remain soft and pliable, but only the porosity of the cuticle permits moisture to be absorbed or dried out.

An understanding of the relationship between the cuticle and cortex and their individual characteristics is essential to the professional for the purposes of hair analysis and treatment. Examining the condition of the cuticle can help the professional to reach probable conclusions concerning the porosity, moisture content, and texture of the hair.

Although we cannot directly view the cortex during hair analysis, the information gained from observing the cuticle, combined with additional analysis testing, such as stretching the hair, redirecting the hair when combing, and by simple touch, provide other probable conclusions. It is the combination of these conclusions that will guide us in product choice, chemical options, and hair design.

Two factors of hair structure that affect the process of hair removal are diameter and elasticity. The diameter must be considered when selecting the size needle to be used and the elasticity indicates the level of moisture, a certain amount of which is required for effective treatment.

The professional must know what should and shouldn't be done to the cuticle and cortex of the hair to avoid permanent damage. Curling, roller setting, and all forms of hairstyling produce artificial or physical changes in the structure of the cortex. Permanent wave solutions, relaxers, and other chemical applications produce chemical changes in the structure of the cortex.

The inherent responsibility that goes along with this knowledge requires the professional to be conscientious in the performance of services and chemical applications.

Medulla

The medulla is the central layer of the hair. It is made up of a column of cells, either two or four rows wide.

The medulla is not always a continuous part of the hair; rather, it is frequently broken or even entirely absent from the hair shaft. This condition is often found in hair and it is suspected that the state of health and the taking of certain medicines have a direct bearing on it.

The purpose or function of the medulla is unknown. Hair does not seem to suffer when it is missing, although it may serve as a channel for nutrients and waste products from the papilla. The medulla has a sponge-like structure made of soft keratin, whereas the cuticle and cortex are formed of hard keratin. Pigment of the hair is often found in this layer as well. (See Figure 2–6.)

NOTE: Hair has no power of self-repair, as opposed to the skin.

Hair Growth and the Nature of Protein

In order to truly understand the complexity of hair growth, we must possess a thorough comprehension of the properties involved in hair formation. Since hair is composed of hard keratin, which is a protein, it is essential to understand the nature of protein. Proteins are complicated organic compounds that are essential for life and contain the elements of carbon, hydrogen, oxygen, and nitrogen. Proteins fall into one of three categories—simple, complex, or fiber proteins.

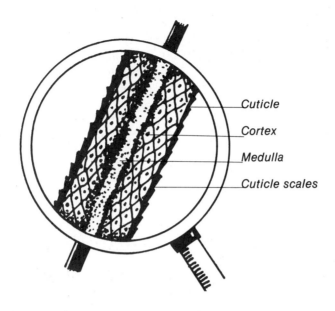

Figure 2–6   Mangification of a cross section of hair

Amino acids are the basic building blocks of proteins, and about 22 types are known to science. Cystine and cysteine are two amino acids of particular interest to stylists. Simple proteins, such as may be found in most food groups, are joined end-on-end by chemical bonds called peptide or end-bonds. The amino acids are joined together in a definite order, and the arrangements of the individual amino acids, chemically joined together by peptide bonds, are called polypeptides. These polypeptides then may form long, coiled chains, containing many hundreds of amino acids. Simple proteins, such as may be found in milk, eggs, fish, and some meats, are water soluble and are easily broken down in the body's digestive system.

Complex proteins form when adjacent spirals of polypeptides are cross-linked by other bonds. The strongest link occurs when sulphur-containing amino acids (such as cystine and cysteine) align opposite to one another on adjacent polypeptide chains. Cystine or sulphur bonds give added strength to the properties of the protein, and the cross-bonds give it a tougher texture. Protein-splitting enzymes (secreted by the digestive system) are required to split the peptide bonds in order to release the amino acids of the protein. These amino acids are water soluble and can be easily absorbed by the body.

Fiber proteins are in the class of proteins that cannot be broken down and consist of countless numbers of polypeptide chains that are twisted into long fibers. Moisture is required to lubricate the polypeptide chains to allow flexibility and pliability. Fiber proteins possess exceptional numbers of cross-bonds: so many that the cross-bonds account for half the weight of the fiber protein. Examples of fiber proteins are human and animal hair, silk, and the horns of some animals. Although the keratin of human hair is a protein, it cannot be formed by consuming other fiber proteins since they are not digestible to humans. The amino acids needed for the formation of hair can only come from edible proteins, and these must be especially rich in sulphur to supply the cross-bonds necessary for fiber proteins. (See Figure 2–7.)

NOTE: Hair has more cross-bonds than any other protein.

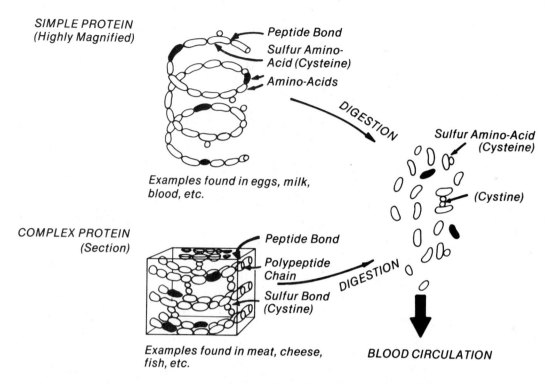

SIMPLE PROTEIN
(Highly Magnified)

Peptide Bond

Sulfur Amino-
Acid (Cysteine)

Amino-Acids

DIGESTION

Examples found in eggs, milk,
blood, etc.

Sulfur Amino-Acid
(Cysteine)

(Cystine)

COMPLEX PROTEIN
(Section)

Peptide Bond

Polypeptide
Chain

DIGESTION

Sulfur Bond
(Cystine)

Examples found in meat, cheese,
fish, etc.

BLOOD CIRCULATION

Figure 2–7   The structure of simple and complex proteins

Bonds of the Hair Cortex

End-Bonds or Peptide Bonds   Peptide bonds are chemical bonds that join the amino acids in a chain. They are the strongest bonds in the cortex. When weakened or damaged through chemical abuse, the bonds break and hair may break off.

Sulphur or Cystine Bonds   The end-bonds hold the long chains of amino acids together end-to-end, but the sulphur or cystine bonds join the chains of the peptide bonds together horizontally, like the rungs of a ladder. These are called cross-bonds, and they supply hair with its tensile strength and shape.

When hair has been processed by certain chemicals, such as waving and relaxing solutions, the amino acid cystine changes to cysteine. The neutralizing process of such solutions cause the cysteine to revert back to cystine. Some agents that will break sulphur bonds are ammonium thioglycolate (waving solutions) and sodium hydroxide (chemical hair relaxers). Agents that will re-form sulphur bonds are permanent wave neutralizer, hydrogen peroxide, and oxygen from the air. All of these agents are considered oxidizers.

NOTE: Cystine bonds are also known as disulfide bonds.

Hydrogen Bonds   Although very weak in singular structure, hydrogen bonds (H-bonds) are the most numerous bonds in the hair. They are also a type of cross-bond that helps the sulphur bond keep the parallel chains of amino acids together. The H-bond is considered a physical rather than a chemical bond because it is only involved with physical changes that take place in the hair. These changes include setting, waving, and curling. Agents that will break hydrogen bonds are water, dilute (less concentrated) alkali, and neutral or acid lotions. Drying (air) and dilute acids will reform hydrogen bonds.

Free Amino Acids Between the chains of keratin in the cortex are free amino acids which hold the moisture within the cortex at the desirable level of 10 percent. Together with sebum, they function as moisturizers or moisture retainers.

Salt Bonds Salt bonds and several other bonds, such as carbon and nitrogen bonds, occur between the polypeptide chains but are not as important as the sulphur and hydrogen bonds, except in the case of an unusual reaction to chemical treatment of the hair.

When performing chemical services, the professional is concerned with the peptide-peptide, sulphur and hydrogen bonds of the hair. When end-bonds (peptides) are broken through chemical abuse, there is no way of re-forming them. Once serious damage has occurred, the only option is to wait until that section of hair grows out to a sufficient length to be trimmed off.

The importance of the sulphur bonds originates from the fact that these bonds supply the hair with its strength and, thus, provide some resistance to solutions and products. Ultimately, of course, the sulphur bonds can be broken with permanent wave and chemical relaxing formulations. A good example of the effect of the sulphur bond content in hair is seen when chemically processing red hair. Red hair contains up to 8 percent sulphur, compared to average hair, which contains 4 to 5 percent sulphur. It is the additional 3 to 4 percent of additional sulphur found in red hair that makes it more resistant to chemical processes, especially permanent waving.

It is also important to keep in mind that it is the breaking of the sulphur bonds during chemical applications that causes softening of the hair, and that the reformation of the sulphur bonds with neutralizing agents results in the hair hardening. Chemical processing causes a permanent chemical change in the structure of the hair.

Hydrogen bonds, on the other hand, can be rearranged with water, setting lotions, or heat. Wet hairstyling, blow-drying, and therm styling are some of the ways in which hydrogen bonds can be broken and re-formed. The performance of these services results in a temporary physical change in the hair structure.

Formation of Hard Keratin in Hair

The cycles of hair growth are known as anagen, catagen, and telogen. (See Figure 2–8.)

Anagen Stage

The formation of hair begins with the digestion of proteins in the diet, where they are broken down to release amino acids into the blood. These amino acids eventually reach the blood capillaries in each papilla and the follicle cells surrounding the

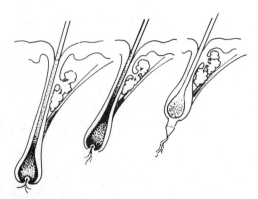

Figure 2-8   The three stages of follicle development: anagen, catagen, and telogen

terminal matrix. The wall of the blood capillary has minute cracks through which fluids are constantly seeping. This bathes the cells with amino acids and provides a food supply. The cell fluids then reach the outer layer of the papilla—a layer of special cells that is part of the epidermis and contacts the germinal matrix. As the germinal matrix forms new cells by continual cell division, the older cells are slowly pushed up the follicle. When first formed, these new cells are similar to those of the germinal matrix. These cells contain a nucleus and a well-defined cell membrane and are 75 percent water. The hair bulb stretchs out into the follicle during this first phase of the anagen stage in the formation of hair.

Phase two of the anlagen stage (when hard keratin is being synthesized in the follicle) begins when the cells moving up the follicle change in appearance from the soft and liquid structure to a harder, dryer look. This metamorphosis occurs by the time the cells have traveled approximately a third of the way up the follicle. The older cells, now located even further up the follicle, will have become part of the cortex layer of the hair, in which the nucleus dies and the cell wall (or membrane) disappears. The contents of the former cells shrink in volume as the water is removed to a much lower level than in the hair bulb (finally down to 10 percent in the mature hair).

In the first formed cells of the cortex, next to the germ layer of the papilla, the amino acids are scattered throughout the contents of the cell. Gradually they join together to form the hard keratin type of chains of amino acids. Then, as the cell walls disappear (in the zone of keratinization), these chains link up crosswise with chains of adjacent cells to form a spiral. The result is a long fiber. In the hair cortex, large numbers of cystine or sulphur cross-bonds join these parallel polypeptide chains together. As the moisture level drops, other bonds, called hydrogen or physical bonds, gradually appear.

Keratinization of the Cuticle   The hard keratin of the cuticle forms in a different manner than the cortex, since it makes a loose, scaly covering around the hair. Consequently, the hard keratin of the cuticle has few of the features of the cortex. The cells in the cuticle layer also lose moisture and become harder and scalier but, unlike those cells in the cortex, they remain somewhat separated.

Mature Hair Fiber

The mature hair fiber has reached the upper extent of the zone of keratinization. The amino acids from the germ layer are fully converted to keratin, and all visible signs of the original cells are gone. Special enzymes can separate these cells, which show as elongated structures.

However, the normal cortex is made of countless billions of long polypeptide chains arranged in a characteristic fiber. The polypeptide chains are joined together by large numbers of cross-bonds. Both sulphur and hydrogen bonds form links that give the polypeptide chains a very strong arrangement.

Catagen Phase

After a period of growth, the catagen phase will begin. The length of time of the growth will depend on many factors such as age, sex, and hormone distribution. The papilla first separates from the bulb at the hair root. Nourishment is then decreased, and the production of germinal cells slows. The follicle walls begin to shrink and to dehydrate.

This phase is usually very brief, and sometimes a new hair can form even while the old hair is still in the follicle. These old hairs are commonly called bed hairs or club hairs.

Telogen

When the catagen stage is complete, the follicle usually rests until it is stimulated to begin a new anagen cycle. This intermediate resting phase is called the telogen stage.

When performing electrolysis treatments, the professional should strive to treat the unwanted hair growth during the anagen stage because in addition to the hair being straight and closer to the skin surface, giving better accessibility, the hair bulb is still in close proximity to the papilla, which can then be permanently destroyed during the treatment. The success rate of electrology is lowered by the amount of hairs that are treated during the telogen stage since the hair is already detached from the papilla and the lower portion of the follicle will not be destroyed.

The telogen stage of hair growth can be determined by examining an epilated hair for evidence of an attached club-shaped bulb and a shriveled appearance of the hair that was inside the follicle.

The importance of maintaining regular appointments should be impressed on clients to assure successful treatments.

In conclusion, it is apparent why a through understanding of the structure of the hair and the many situations in which the knowledge may be applied, is of vital importance to the beauty industry professional. There exists an inherent responsibility that accompanies this knowledge, for it requires the application of qualified skills, accurate analysis and judgment, and adherence to an ethical standard of performance.

2

Fill in the Blank

1. Understanding the physiology and histology of hair is of vital importance to _____

   _____ .

2. Name two services professionals perform that may influence the nature of hair.

   1. _____

   2. _____

3. Hair growth is enabled by the development of _____ into the dermis.

4. Lanugo and vellus hair are considered to be _____ types.

5. Hair that is more stiff and bristly is known as _____ .

6. _____ or _____ hair is found on the scalp.

7. Two distinctive characteristics used to categorize the three main types of hair are:

   1. _____

   2. _____

8. List four changes in the body that may result in different types of hair growth.

   1. _____   3. _____

   2. _____   4. _____

9. Identify the main hair types—primary, secondary, and tertiary—with the following characteristics.

   _____ 1. A probable increase in thickness and number with age.

   _____ 2. Lack of medulla.

   _____ 3. A large medulla in many cases.

   _____ 4. Hair found on the scalp.

   _____ 5. May appear as multiple hairs.

   _____ 6. Lacks pigment.

   _____ 7. A curved shape in many cases.

_____ 8. Lacks an arrector pili muscle.

_____ 9. The follicles lie at angles.

_____ 10. Aids in the evaporation of perspiration.

_____ 11. More sensitive to touch than scalp hair.

_____ 12. May be found in beards and mustaches.

_____ 13. Hairs not lost in the balding process.

_____ 14. Pigmented hair.

_____ 15. May possess a natural wave.

_____ 16. Has at least one sebaceous gland and an arrector pili muscle.

10. The _____ surrounds the hair root.

11. The hair follicle is made up of an _____ sheath and an _____ sheath.

12. The external root sheath is a downward continuation of the _____.

13. The stratum basale is part of the _____.

14. The stratum basale is a single layer of _____ capable of _____.

15. A terminal layer at the base of the hair bulb is called the _____.

16. The _____ is formed from the cells of the matrix.

17. The internal root sheath separates the _____ from the _____.

18. Diagram of a section of the scalp. Identify and insert the parts of the skin below.

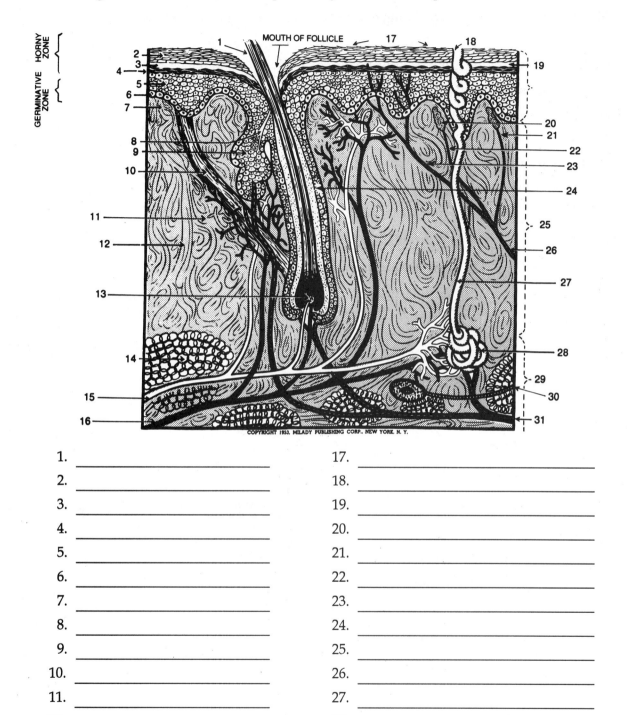

1. _____
2. _____
3. _____
4. _____
5. _____
6. _____
7. _____
8. _____
9. _____
10. _____
11. _____
12. _____
13. _____
14. _____
15. _____
16. _____

17. _____
18. _____
19. _____
20. _____
21. _____
22. _____
23. _____
24. _____
25. _____
26. _____
27. _____
28. _____
29. _____
30. _____
31. _____

19. Follicle groups contain _____ to _____ hairs each.

20. The effect of two hairs appearing to grow from the same follicle is known as _____ _____.

21. The structure of the hair root includes the _____ and the _____.

22. Melanin is produced by special cells in the _____.

23. A cone-shaped elevation of loose, connective tissue is the _____.

24. Cells in the germinal matrix are able to change food sources into _____.

25. List four substances that make up sebum:
    1. _____   3. _____
    2. _____   4. _____

26. The color of blackheads is due to _____ and _____.

27. Perspiration is a mixture of _____, _____, _____, _____, _____, _____, _____, _____, and _____.

28. _____ are the building blocks of all protein.

29. The function of the cuticle is to protect the _____ from _____.

30. The _____ is responsible for most of the behavior of human hair.

31. List eight physical properties of the cortex.
    1. _____   5. _____
    2. _____   6. _____
    3. _____   7. _____
    4. _____   8. _____

32. _____ and _____ allow the hair to be stretched and ensure its return to a normal position.

33. The pliability of hair depends on a combination of the _____ of hair.

34. The most influencing factors of follicle design are _____ and _____ in nature.

35. The mass of hair is due to the _____ in the cortex.

36. A. Name the two main parts of the hair:
    1. _____
    2. _____

    B. Using numbers 1 and 2 from question 36A above, match them with the following characteristics.
    _____ 1. Will resist wear or friction but has no strength.
    _____ 2. Has great strength but cannot resist wear or friction.
    _____ 3. Holds together very well but is easily damaged.

_____ 4. Protects but does not hold together.

_____ 5. Allows waving and setting to take place.

_____ 6. Has the ability to be waved or set.

_____ 7. Has elastic properties.

_____ 8. Allows the hair to be stretched.

_____ 9. Permits moisture to be absorbed or dried out.

_____ 10. Requires moisture in order to remain soft and pliable.

37. The _____ may serve as a channel for nutrients and waste products from the papilla.

38. The medulla has a sponge-like structure made of _____ .

39. List four elements contained in protein essential for life.

    1. _____   3. _____

    2. _____   4. _____

40. List three classifications of proteins.

    1. _____   3. _____

    2. _____

41. Amino acids joined end-to-end by chemical bonds are known as _____ or

    _____ .

42. Strings of amino acids joined together by peptide bonds are called _____ .

43. _____ form when adjacent spirals of polypeptides are cross-linked by other bonds.

44. _____ or _____ provide added strength to the protein.

45. _____ cannot be broken down.

46. Give four examples of fiber proteins.

    1. _____   3. _____

    2. _____   4. _____

47. Edible proteins must be rich in _____ to supply the cross-bonds necessary for fiber proteins.

48. _____ has more cross-bonds than any other protein.

49. _____ are the strongest bonds in the cortex.

50. _____ or _____ are the cross-bonds in hair.

51. Sulphur bonds are also known as _____ or _____ .

52. The sulphur bonds supply the hair with _____ and shape.

53. Some chemicals will change the amino acid cystine to _____ .

54. The _____ process will revert cysteine back to cystine.

55. Give two chemical agents that will break sulphur bonds.

    1. _____   2. _____

56. List three agents that will re-form sulphur bonds.

    1. _____   3. _____

    2. _____

57. Hydrogen bonds are the most _____ bonds in the hair.

58. Cross-bonds that help the sulphur bonds to keep the chains of amino-acids together are known as _____.

59. Hydrogen bonds are considered to be _____.

60. List four agents that will break hydrogen bonds.

    1. _____   3. _____

    2. _____   4. _____

61. Name two agents that will reform hydrogen bonds.

    1. _____   2. _____

62. Free amino-acids are located _____ in the cortex.

63. _____ maintain moisture at a desirable level in the cortex.

64. _____ and _____ bonds also occur between the polypeptide chains.

65. The three stages of hair growth are _____, _____, and _____.

66. The anagen stage has two phases, the _____ and the _____.

67. Hard keratin is synthesized in the _____.

68. Bed hairs or club hairs are found during the _____ stage.

69. During the catagen stage, the _____ separates from the _____ at the hair root.

70. The resting stage is known as the _____ stage.

3

The Body Framework

Introduction to the Skeletal System

The skeletal system is the bony framework of the body (composed of 206 individual bones in the adult body). There are five specific functions of the skeletal system, which are described below:

1. Supports the body structures and provides shape to the body.
2. Protects the soft and delicate internal organs, such as the brain, heart, lungs, and spinal cord.
3. Provides the movement and anchorage of muscles (muscles that are attached to the skeleton are called skeletal muscles).
4. Provides storage for minerals like calcium and phosphorous and releases the necessary amounts of minerals when needed to maintain homeostasis (maintenence of optimal internal environmental conditions).
5. Performs hemopoiesis whereby the red marrow of the bone is the site of blood cell formation.

Bone Types

Bones are classified as one of four types, depending on their form. Long bones are located in the upper and lower arms and legs. The wrist and ankle bones are short bones which appear club-like in shape. Irregular bones are represented by bones of the spinal column, and flat bones are seen in the skull and the ribs.

Joints

The degree of movement at a joint is determined by bone shape and joint structure. **Joints** are points of contact between two bones which are classified into three main types according to the degree of movement. They are diarthroses, or movable joints; amphiarthroses, or partially movable joints; and synarthroses, or immovable joints. (See Figure 3–1.)

Most of the joints of the body are **diarthroses (deye-are-THROH-sees)**. They tend to have the identical structures and to consist of three main parts: articular cartilage, a bursa (joint capsule), and a synovial (joint) cavity.

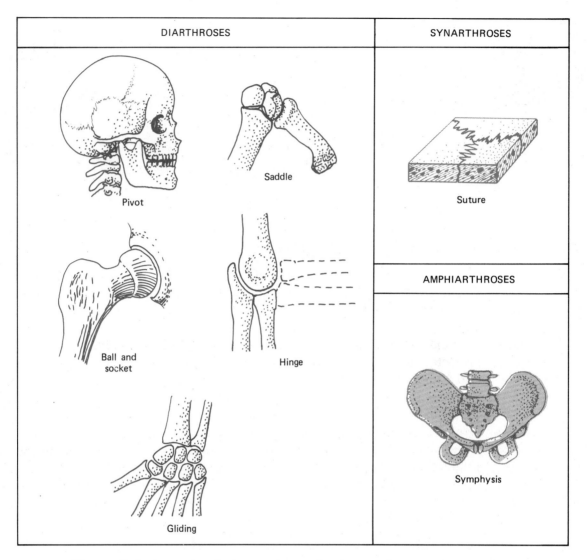

Figure 3-1 Joints classified according to the degree of movement permitted

When two movable bones meet at a joint, the surfaces do not touch but rather are covered with a cap of cartilage called articular cartilage which helps absorb jolts. The articular capsule is a tough, fibrous connective tissue that encloses two articular surfaces of the bone. Lining the articular capsule is the synovial membrane which secretes (into an area between two articular cartilages) a lubricating substance known as **synovial (sih-NOH-vee-all) fluid** which reduces the friction of joint movement.

With age, the joints may undergo degenerative changes because the synovial fluid is not secreted as adequately and the articular cartilage surfaces of the bone ends become ossified. This results in excess bone growths along the joint edges, which tends to stiffen joints, causing inflammation, pain, and decreases in mobility, which can lead to different types of arthritis (of which the professional ought to be aware). See the section titled "Disorders of the Bones and Joints," later in this chapter, for further information.

Types of Diarthroses Joints

Type	Characteristics	Example
Ball and socket joints	Allows greatest freedom movement; one bone is ball-shaped and fits into the concave socket of another bone.	Shoulders and hips.
Hinge joints	Move in one direction or plane.	Knees, elbows, outer joints of fingers.
Pivot joints	Have an extension that rotates in a second, arch-long shaped bone; allow the head to rotate.	Long bones of the forearm; wrist, and ankle; joint between first and second cervical vertebra in neck.
Gliding joints	Nearly flat surfaces that glide across each other; they enable the torso to bend back and forth and to rotate.	Vertebrae of the spine.

The **amphiarthroses (am-fee-are-THROH-sees)** are partially movable joints that have cartilage between their articular surfaces. Examples are the attchement of ribs to the spine and symphysis and the joint between the two pubic bones.

Synarthroses (sin-are-THROH-sees) are immovable joints connected by tough, fibrous connective tissue. They are found in the adult cranium, where the bones are fused together in a joint that forms a protective covering for the brain.

Joints are also bound together by **ligaments (LIG-ah-ments)**, which are fibrous bands that connect bones and cartilages and serve as support for muscles.

Tendons are the fibrous cords that connect muscles to bones.

Types of Motion

As can be seen in Figure 3–2 joints can move in many directions.

Flexion (FLEK-shun) is the act of bending forward, as when the forearm or fingers are bent or flexed.

Extension means to straighten the forearm or fingers.

Abduction is the movement of an extremity away from the midline.

Adduction is movement toward the midline.

A **rotation** movement allows a bone to move around one central axis. Two rotation movements are pronation (the forearm turns the hand so that the palm is downward) and supination (the palm is turned upward).

Structure and Formation of Bone

Bones are composed of mature bone cells called osteocytes and consist of 35 percent organic material and 65 percent inorganic material. The organic portion of bone

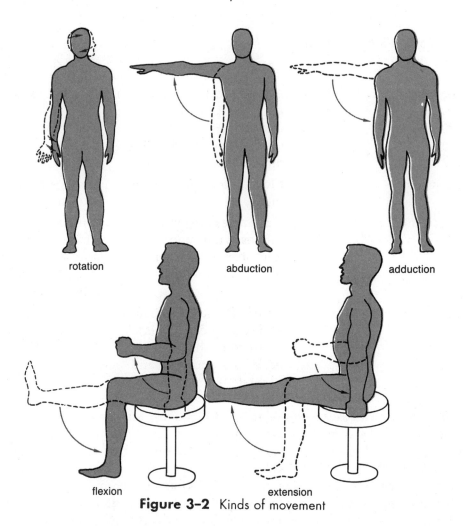

rotation   abduction   adduction

flexion   extension

Figure 3-2 Kinds of movement

stems from a protein called bone collagen, a fibrous matrial that gives bone a certain degree of flexibility. The inorganic ratio of bone is made from mineral salts such as calcium phosphate, calcium cabonate, calcium fluoride, magnesium phosphate, sodium oxide, and sodium chloride, which provide strength and durability.

Bone Formation

The embryonic skeleton is initially composed of collagenous protein fibers secreted by embryonic cells, followed by the deposit of cartilage between the fibers. At this stage, the embryonic skeleton consists of collagenous protein fibers and clear (hyaline) cartilage. During the eighth week of development, mineral matter starts to replace previously formed cartilage (the process of ossification), creating bone.

Structure

Long bones are composed of a shaft that is a hollow cylinder of hard, compact bone. This allows the bone to be strong and hard yet light enough for movement. In the center of the shaft is the medullary canal, which is filled with yellow bone marrow, consisting mostly of fat cells. The marrow also contains blood vessels and cells that form leukocytes (white blood cells), and it acts as a fat storage center. The endosteum is the lining of the marrow canal, which keeps the cavity intact.

The ends of the long bones contain red marrow where some red blood cells (erythrocytes) and some white blood cells are made. The outside of the bone is covered with the periosteum, a fibrous tissue containing blood vessels, lymph vessels, and nerves, which is necessary for bone growth, repair, and nutrition.

Bones grow in length and ossify from the center of the shaft (diaphysis) toward the ends (epiphysis). As ossification occurs in the growth zone, causing the bone to lengthen, it causes the ends of the bone to grow away from the middle of the shaft. The length of a bone shaft continues to grow until all the epiphyseal cartilage is ossified. The average growth in females continues until about 18 years, and in males, to 20 or 21 years. New bone growth in the case of breaks or fractures can occur at any time, as bone cells near the site of an injury will become active.

Parts of the Skeleton

The skeletal system is comprised of two main parts. The axial skeleton consists of the skull, spinal column, ribs, breastbone, and hyoid bone (a U-shaped bone in the neck to which the tongue is attached). The appendicular skeleton includes the upper extremities—the shoulder girdles, arms, wrists and hands, and the lower extremities—the hip girdle, legs, ankles, and feet. (See Figure 3–3.)

Axial Skeleton

The skull is composed of the cranium and facial bones which house and protect the brain and guard and support the eyes, ears, nose, and mouth, respectively. Some facial bones, such as the nasal bones, are made of bone and cartilage. The bridge of the nose is bone, while the lower part is cartilage.

There are 22 bones in the skull—8 in the cranium and 14 in the facial areas. (See Figure 3–4.)

> **NOTE:** The skull contains large spaces (cavities) within the facial bones. Refered to as paranasal sinuses, they are lined with mucous membranes. When a person suffers from a cold, hayfever, or allergies, the membranes become inflamed and swollen, resulting in excess mucus. This may lead to sinus pain and a "stuffy" sensation.

Spine The spine or vertebral column is strong and flexible, providing support for the head and a point of attachment for the ribs. Most important, the spine encloses and protects the spinal cord of the nervous system.

Vertebrae are small bones that are separated from each other by pads of cartilage tissue called intervertebral disks. Within the developing embryo there are 33 separate vertebrae. However, before birth several will fuse together, leaving 26. Figure 3–5, page 64, depicts a lateral and dorsal view of the vertebrae of the spine.

The spine is curved rather than straight, thus providing more strength. Its shape also provides the proper balance for the human bipedal (two-footed) posture.

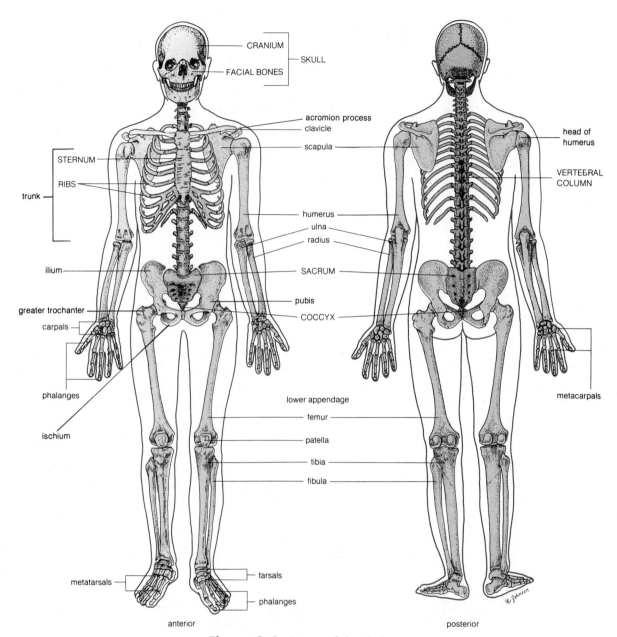

Figure 3-3 Bones of the skeleton

NOTE: Before birth, the thoracic and sacral regions are convex curves. As the infant learns to hold up its head, the cervical region becomes concave, and when the child learns to stand, the lumbar area also becomes concave. This completes the four curves of a normal, adult human spine.

Ribs and Sternum The thoracic vertebrae, ribs, and sternum protect the thoracic area of the body. The breastbone, or sternum, is divided into three parts: the upper region (manubrium), the body, and a lower part known as the xiphoid process. The collar bones (clavicles) are attached by means of ligaments to the upper region of the sternum. The human body contains 12 pairs of ribs. The first 7 pairs are joined by costal cartilages directly to the sternum and are known as true ribs. The next 3 pairs are called

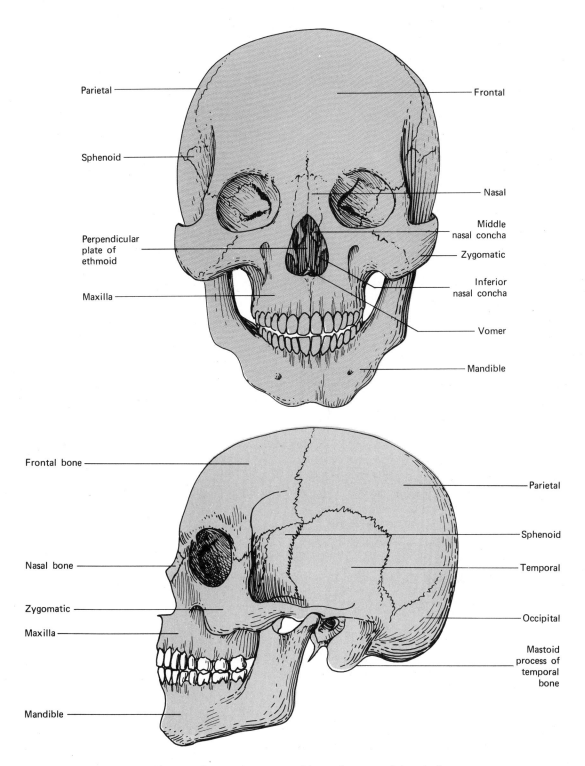

Figure 3–4 Anterior and lateral views of the skull

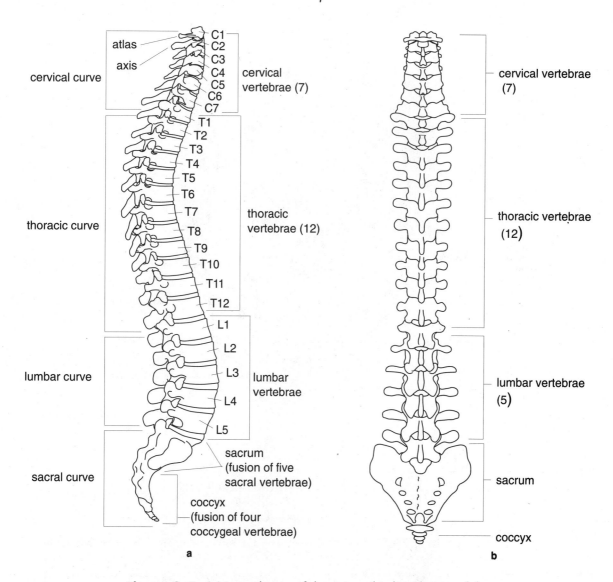

Figure 3-5 (a) Lateral view of the spine; (b) dorsal view of the spine

false ribs because their costal cartilages are attached to the seventh rib instead of directly to the sternum. The last 2 pairs of ribs are not connected to either the costal cartilages nor the sternum and are therefore called floating ribs.

Appendicular Skeleton

The appendicular skeleton includes the 126 bones of the upper and lower extremities, which include the body structures of the shoulder girdle, arms, hands, pelvic girdle, upper legs, lower legs, ankles, and feet.

The shoulder girdle consists of two curved clavicles and two triangular scapulae (shoulder bones). The scapulae provide a place of attachment for the arms and permit the attachment of muscles for arm movement. The clavicles help brace the shoulders and prevent excessive forward motion.

The bone structure of the arm consists of the humerus in the upper arm and the

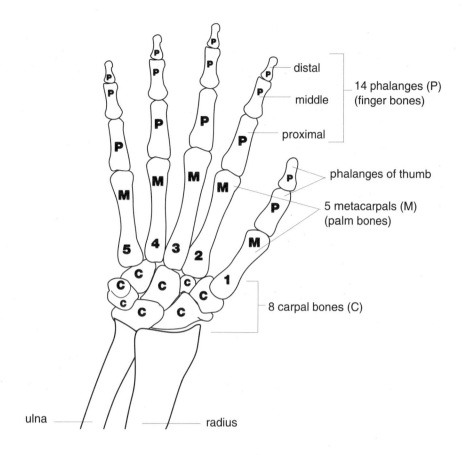

Figure 3–6 Diagram showing the 27 bones of the right hand—dorsal view

radius and ulna in the forearm. The humerus is the second largest bone in the body and is attached to the scapula by muscles (biceps and triceps) and ligaments. In the forearm, the radius runs up the thumb side and provides rotation of the ulna. This characteristic permits the hand to rotate freely and with great flexibility. The ulna is far more limited in motion and, at its upper end, it forms the elbow.

The wrist bone (ossa carpi) consists of eight small bones arranged in two rows that are held together by ligments which allow mobility and flexion.

The hand is composed of two parts: 5 metacarpal bones and 14 phalanges. Each finger, except for the thumb, has 3 phalanges. Hinge joints between these bones allow the fingers to be bent easily. (See Figure 3–6.)

The pelvic girdle serves as area of attachment for the bones and muscles of   leg, in addition to providing support for the soft organs of the lower abdominal region. The pelvic bones of a female are wider, lighter, and smoother than those of males, mostly to accommodate the process of childbirth.

The upper leg contains the thigh bone, or femur, which is the longest and strongest bone in the body. The lower leg consists of the tibia, the largest of the lower leg bones, and the fibula, which is the slender bone on the outside edge of the lower leg. The patella, or kneecap, is a flat, triangular, sesamoid bone that is found in front of the knee joint. Surrounding the patella are four bursae, which cushion the joint.

The ankle (tarsus) contains 7 tarsal bones, which provide a connection between the foot and leg bones. Ankle movement is a silding motion that allowes the foot to extend and flex when walking.

The foot has five metatarsal bones, which are somewhat comparable to the metacarpals of the hand. However, the metatarsal and tarsal bones are arranged to form two arches. The longitudinal arch runs from the heel to the points of connection of the metatarsals and the phalanges (toe bones). The transverse arch lies perpendicular to the longitudiinal arch in the metatarsal region. Arches strengthen the foot and provide flexibility and a "spring" to the step. (See Figure 3–7.)

> *In some cases, arches may fall due to weak foot ligaments and tendons. The downward pressure of the weight of the body slowly flattens them, causing "fallen arches" or "flatfeet." Factors that may lead to this conditon include improper prenatal nutrition, dietary or hormonal imbalances, fatigue, being overweight, poor posture, and shoes that do not fit properly. Professionals should be consciously aware of all these factors, especially in the choice of shoes and the practicing of correct posture in the workplace in order to prevent fallen arches. For the professional engaged in providing pedicures and massage to to clients, use the client consultation aspect of the service and observe whether this condition is present (be aware that pain may also be present). As with other massage services, talk with your client to determine the most comfortable pressure level.*

The toes are similar in composition to the fingers. There are three phalanges in each with the exception of the big toe which, like the thumb, has only two.

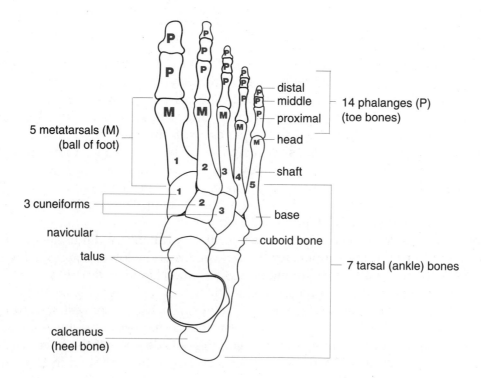

Figure 3–7 Dorsal view of the right foot and its 26 bones

Disorders of the Bones and Joints

Fractures and breaks are the most common injuries to bones and result in swelling and bleeding tissues. The process of restoring a fractured bone to its original position is called reduction. A cast is applied to hold the fracture in place and immobile while healing occurs.

Common Types of Fractures

- Closed—the bone is broken but the broken ends do not pierce the skin.
- Open—the most serious type of fracture, in which the broken bone ends pierce through the skin, forming an external wound, which is subject to infection.
- Greenstick—the simplest type of fracture, in which the bone is partially bent but does not completely separate. These fractures are common among children due to the amount of flexible cartilage in their bones.
- Comminuted—in this case, the bone is splintered or broken into many pieces which can become embedded in the surrounding tissue.

Bone and Joint Injuries

1. Dislocation—the bone is displaced from its proper position in a joint, which may result in tearing or stretching of ligaments. Return of the bone to its proper position is necessary, followed by rest for the ligaments to heal.
2. Sprain—an injury to a joint caused by a sudden or unusual motion, such as "turning" or "twisting" the ankle. The ligaments may be torn from their attachments to the bones or torn crosswise, but the joint is not dislocated. Sprains are accompanied by rapid swelling and acute pain in the area, and treatment consists of supporting the joint (with adhesive strapping or an elasticized bandage) until the ligaments heal.
3. Ankylosis—the abnormal immobility and consolidation of a joint as a result of the bones having fused solid.
4. Arthritis—an inflammatory condition of one or more joints, accompanied by pain and, often, changes in bone position. The most common types are rheumatoid arthritis, osteoarthritis, and gouty arthritis.
   a. Rheumatoid arthritis is a chronic systemic disease affecting the connective tissue and joints. It results in acute inflammation of the connective tissue, thickening of the synovial membrane, and ankylosis of the joints. The pain that accompanies this conditon causes muscle spasms that may lead to deformities in the joints. Additionally, the cartilage that separates the joints will degenerate and hard calcium will begin to fill the spaces. As joints become stiff and immobile, the attached muscles begin to atrophy (wasting away of tissue). Rheumatoid arthritis usually affects the entire body.
   b. Osteoarthritis—a degenerative joint disease in which the cartilage at the ends of the bones progressively wears down, distorting the joint position. The surrounding tendons, ligaments, and muscles become weaker, and the joint becomes painful, stiff and deformed. Pain is usually present, but there is generally little or no swelling and disablement is minimal. Osteoarthritis rarely develops before age 40; it is typically hereditary and affects more women than men.

c. Gouty arthritis is caused by a faulty uric acid metabolism and occurs more often in overweight individuals and those who regularly indulge in rich foods and alcohol. Uric acid crystals deposit in the joints, especially those of the big toe. Men tend to suffer from gouty arthritis more often than women.

Massage should not be performed on inflamed and painful areas of the body. However, a gentle massage may prove soothing in the surrounding area or in areas that are not inflamed. As a professional, you may suggest that a client with arthritis discuss with his or her physician, and/or a nutritionist, the possible benefits of vitamins, diets, and exercises to alleviate pain and the further deterioration of the joints. For instance, it is thought that iron is involved in causing pain, swelling, and joint destruction. Thus, any iron ingested should be consumed naturally from foods and not through vitamin supplements. On the other hand, certain amino acids are thought to have the ability to help remove metals from the system, which may prove beneficial to the arthritic client. Hot tubs and baths may also provide some relief. Although it is not the place of the beauty care professional to diagnosis or prescribe a client's condition, this type of information may certainly be relayed through conversation during a service, providing it is understood that the client should seek a physician's advice in the matter.

---

5. Bunion—a swelling of the bursa (a small sac between parts that move against each other) of the foot, usually of the joint on the big toe, which then becomes adducted. Bunions are usually the result of poorly fitting shoes, poor walking posture, or a hereditary trait.
6. Rickets—a disease of the bones caused by a lack of vitamin D, calcium, and phosphorous, whereby portions of the bone become soft due to lack of calcification, causing such deformities as bowlegs and knock-knees. Sometimes rickets may be caused by an absorption problem resulting from severe allergies, asthma, or colon infections, or through lack of enough natural sunshine.
7. Clubfoot—a congenital malformation that may involve one or both feet.
8. Spina bifida—a congenital condition in which the vertebral column does not develop completely and unite correctly, usually affecting the lumbar and sacral regions.
9. Osteoporosis—a gradual loss of bone mass in both men and women, usually caused by hormonal imbalances. Estrogen deficiency is the usual cause of osteoporosis in women. Preventative treatment includes a diet that is adequate in protein, calcium, vitamins C and D, and exercise.
10. Bursitis—an acute inflammation of the synovial bursa, which cushions a joint during motion. It can be caused by local or systemic inflammation or tension, resulting in formation of calcium deposits which impede the movement of joints.
11. Scoliosis—a lateral (horizontal) curvature of the spine.
12. Subluxation—one of the most common conditions associated with neck injuries, in which a vertebra is displaced from its normal position or range of motion without being completely dislocated. Although whiplash is the usual cause of a subluxated neck, it can also occur through unexpected body movements, blows to the chin or head, or as a result of violent coughing or sneezing.
13. Lumbago—a backache in the lower lumbar region of the spinal column.
14. Neoplasms—various types of tumors that can occur in bone.

Fill in the Blank

1. There are _____ individual bones in the body.

2. The functions of the skeletal system are to _____ the _____,
   provide _____ to the body, protect _____, provide _____
   and _____ of muscles, provide _____ storage, and to provide the site
   of _____ formation.

3. The four types of bones are _____ bones, _____ bones, _____ bones
   and _____ bones.

4. _____ are points of contact between two bones.

5. The degree of movement in a joint is determined by _____ and _____
   _____ .

6. Joints are classified according to the _____ of _____ .

7. Most of the joints of the body are classified as _____ .

8. The surfaces of two movable bones are covered with a cap of _____ .

9. _____ lubricates the cartilages and reduces the friction of joint movement.

10. With age, the cartilage surfaces may become _____ , which leads to different types
    of _____ .

11–14 Provide one example of each type of diarthroses joint.

11. Ball and socket   _____

12. Hinge   _____

13. Pivot   _____ long bones for wrist or ankle, or be-
                             tween first and second vertebrae in neck

14. Gliding   _____ of the spine

15. _____ are fibrous bands that connect bones and cartilage.

16. _____ are fibrous cords that connect muscles to bones.

17. _____ is the act of bending forward.

18. _____ means to straighten.

19. A _____ allows a bone to move around one central axis.

20. Bones consist of _____ material and _____ material.

21. The organic portion of bone consists of a protein called _____ .

22. The inorganic portion of bone consists of _____ .

23. Blood vessels and cells in the marrow of bones form leukocytes, or _____ cells.

24. Erythrocytes is the term used for _____ cells.

25. Bones grow and ossify from the _____ to the _____ .

26. The skeletal system is comprised of the _____ skeleton and the _____ skeleton.

27. The skull is composed of the _____ and _____ bones.

28. There are _____ bones in the cranium and _____ bones in the facial areas.

29. The paranasal sinuses are lined with _____ .

30. _____ , _____ , or _____ may swell and inflame the paranasal sinuses.

31. The most important function of the spine is that it _____ and _____ the spinal cord.

32. The spine also provides the _____ for human posture.

33. The human body contains _____ pairs of ribs.

34. The _____ help brace the shoulders and prevent excessive forward motion.

35. The bone structure of the _____ consists of the humerus, radius, and ulna.

36. The _____ is the second largest bone in the body.

37. The _____ provides rotation of the ulna.

38. Rotation of the ulna permits the hand to _____ freely.

39. The wrist bone consists of _____ small bones.

40. The two parts of the hand are _____ bones and _____ .

41. the ankle contains _____ tarsal bones.

42. The foot contains _____ metatarsal bones.

43. _____ strengthen the foot and provide flexibility.

44. The downward pressure of the _____ of the body may cause "fallen arches."

45. The professional should use the _____ and _____ to determine whether a client has fallen arches.

46. _____ may also accompany the fallen arch condition.

47. _____ and _____ are the most common injuries to bones.

48. _____ should not be performed on inflamed or painful areas of the body.

Matching

49–51 Match the following joint classifications with the characteristics.

   amphiarthroses   diarthroses   synarthroses

49. _____ partially movable joint

50. _____ immovable joints

51. _____ movable joints

52–58. Match the following conditions with the appropriate description.

   Arthritis   Bursitis   Closed fracture   Dislocation   Gouty arthritis
   Osteoporosis   Rheumatoid arthritis   Sprain

52. _____ The bone is displaced from its proper position in a joint.

53. _____ The bone is broken but the ends do not pierce the skin.

54. _____ An inflammatory condition of one or more joints accompanied by pain.

55. _____ Caused by a faulty uric acid metabolism.

56. _____ An injury to a joint caused by sudden or unusual motion.

57. _____ A chronic systemic disease affecting the connective tissue and joints.

58. _____ A gradual loss of bone mass, usually caused by hormonal imbalances.

59. _____ An acute inflammation of the synovial bursa, caused by inflammation or tension.

The Muscular System

The ability to move is made possible by the function of contractibility in muscles. Muscle tissue comprises nearly half the total body weight and provides the following functions: allows the body to move from place to place and allows the movement of individual parts of the body, assists in helping to keep the body erect and influences posture, produces most of the body's heat, participates in the movements of the internal organs, and gives the body its characteristic form. The skeleton determines the overall body shape, but the muscles produce the contours.

Types of Muscles

All body movements are determined by the three principal types of muscles—skeletal (striated), smooth (spindle-shaped), and cardiac (nonstriated). Table 4–1 provides a summary of the characteristics of the three principal muscle types.

Attachment of Muscles

All muscles have three characteristics in common—contractibility, extensibility, and elasticity.

Contractibility is a quality possessed by no other body tissue. When a muscle

Table 4-1 Summary of Characteristics of the Three Major Muscle Groups

MUSCLE TYPE	LOCATION	STRUCTURE	FUNCTION
Skeletal muscle (striated, voluntary)	Attached to the skeleton and also located in the wall of the pharynx and esophagus.	A skeletal muscle fiber is long, cylindrical, multinucleated, and contains alternating light and dark striations. Nuclei located at edge of fiber.	Contractions occur voluntarily and may be rapid and forceful.
Smooth muscle (nonstriated, involuntary)	Located in the walls of tubular structures and hollow organs, such as in the digestive tract, urinary bladder, and blood vessels.	A smooth muscle fiber is long and spindle-shaped with no striations.	Contractions occur involuntarily and are rhythmic and slow.
Cardiac (heart) muscle	In the heart	Short, branching fibers with a centrally located nucleus; striations not distinct	Contractions occur involuntarily and are rhythmic and automatic.

shortens or contracts, it reduces the distance between the parts of its contents or the space it surrounds. Hence, the contraction of skeletal muscles that connect a pair of bones brings the attachment points closer together, causing the body to move. When cardiac muscles contract, the area in the heart chambers is reduced, which pumps blood from the heart into the blood vessels. Smooth muscles surround blood vessels and the intestines, which cause the diameter of these tubes to decrease upon contraction. Extensibility is the ability to be stretched, and elasticity, the ability of a muscle to return to its original form or length when relaxed.

In order for muscles to produce movement, they must be attached to bones for leverage, allowing the exertion of force. Muscles are attached to the bones by tendons, while bones are connected by joints. Muscles are attached at both ends to bones, cartilage, ligaments, tendons, skin, and, occasionally, each other. The **origin (OR-ih-jin)** is the part of a skeletal muscle that is attached to a fixed structure or bone which moves least during muscle contraction. The **insertion** is the other end, and is attached to a movable part and moves the most during a muscle contraction. The **belly** is the central area or body of the muscle.

The muscles of the body are arranged in pairs whereby one produces movement in a single direction and the other does so in the opposite direction. The arrangement of two muscles with opposite actions is known as an antagonist pair. For example, one end of the biceps is attached to the scapula and humerus (its origin), and when the biceps contract, these two bones remain stationary. The opposite end of the biceps is attached to the radius of the lower arm (its insertion), and this bone moves upon contraction of the biceps.

Muscle fatigue is caused by an accumulation of lactic acid in the muscles. This may occur during periods of vigorous exercise, when the blood is unable to transport enough oxygen for the complete oxidation of glucose in the muscles. This causes the muscles to contract without oxygen (anaerobically), which hinders muscular contraction, causing muscle fatigue and cramps.

Muscle tone is the condition of a muscle always being slightly contracted and ready to pull. It can be achieved through proper nutrition and regular exercise.

As previously mentioned in Chapter 3, the skeletal muscles are classified into two major muscle groups: the axial muscle group, which consists of the head, face, neck, and trunk muscles, and the appendicular muscle group, which is made up of the extremity muscles.

The muscles of the head control facial expression and the act of mastication (chewing). (See Tables 4–2 and 4–3.)

The muscles of the neck move the head through extension, flexion, and rotation movements. (See Table 4–4.)

The muscles of the upper extremities help move the shoulder (scapula), arm (humerus), forearm, wrist, hand, and fingers. (See Table 4–5.)

The muscles of the trunk control breathing and the movements of the abdomen and the pelvis. (See Table 4–6.)

The muscles of the lower extremities assist in the movement of the thigh (femur), leg, ankle, foot, and toes. (See Table 4–7.)

Table 4-2   Representative Muscles of Facial Expression

MUSCLE	EXPRESSION	LOCATION	FUNCTION
Frontalis	Surprise	On either side of the forehead	Raises eyebrow and wrinkles forehead
Depressor anguli oris	Doubt, disdain, contempt	Found along the side of the chin	Depresses corner of mouth
Orbicularis oris	Doubt, disdain, contempt	Ring-shaped muscle found around the mouth	Compresses and closes the lips
Platysma (broad sheet muscle)	Horror	Broad, thin muscular sheet covering the side of the neck and lower jaw	Draws corners of mouth downward and backward
Zygomaticus major	Laughing or smiling	Extends diagonally upward from corner of mouth	Raises corner of mouth
Nasalis	Muscles of the nose	Found over the nasal bones	Closes and opens the nasal openings
Orbicularis oculi	Sadness	Surrounds the eye orbit underlying the eyebrows	Closes the eyelid and tightens the skin on the forehead

Table 4-3   Representative Muscles of Mastication

MUSCLE	LOCATION	FUNCTION
Masseter	Covers the lateral surface of the ramus (angle) of the mandible	Closes the jaw
Temporalis	Located on the temporal fossa of the skull	Raises the jaw and closes the mouth and draws the jaw backward

Table 4-4   Representative Muscles of the Neck

MUSCLE	LOCATION	FUNCTION
Sternocleidomastoid (two heads)	Large muscles extending diagonally across sides of neck	Flexes head; rotates the head toward opposite side from muscle
Semispinalis capitis	A band of muscle composed of several strips lying along the cervical and thoracic spines.	Extends the head and rotates it to the opposite side
Splenius capitis	Extends diagonally across the posterolateral side of the neck	When both contract, pulls head backward; when only one contracts, rotates head and tips the face upward

Table 4–5   Representative Muscles of the Upper Extremities

MUSCLE	LOCATION	FUNCTION
Trapezius	A large triangular muscle located on upper surface of back	Moves the shoulder; extends the head
Deltoid	A thick triangular muscle that covers the shoulder joint	Abducts the upper arm
Pectoralis major	Anterior part of the chest	Flexes the upper arm and helps to adduct the upper arm
Serratus	Anterior chest	Moves scapula forward and helps to raise the arm
Biceps brachii	Upper arm to radius	Flexes the lower arm
Triceps brachii	Posterior arm to ulna	Extends the lower arm
Extensor and flexor carpi muscle groups	Extends from the anterior and posterior forearm to the hand	Moves the hand
Extensor and flexor digitorum muscle groups	Extends from the anterior and posterior forearm to the fingers	Moves the fingers

Table 4–6   Representative Muscles of the Trunk

MUSCLE	LOCATION	FUNCTION
External intercostals	Found between the ribs	Raises the ribs to help in breathing
Diaphragm	A dome-shaped muscle separating the thoracic and abdominal cavities	Helps to control breathing
Rectus abdominis	Extends from the ribs to the pelvis	Compresses the abdomen
External oblique	Anterior inferior edge of the last eight ribs	Depresses ribs, flexes the spinal column, and compresses the abdominal cavity
Internal oblique	Found directly beneath the external oblique, its fibers running in the opposite direction	Same as above

Exercise and training will alter the size, structure, and strength of a muscle but will not increase the number of muscle fibers. The effects of training on muscular strength are as follows: increase in muscle size, improved antagonistic muscle coordination, and improved functioning in the cortical brain region, where nerve impulses start the

Table 4–7   Representative Muscles of the Lower Extremities

MUSCLE	LOCATION	FUNCTION
Gluteus maximus	Buttocks	Extends femur and rotates it outward
Gluteus medius	Extends from the deep femur to the buttocks	Abducts and rotates the thigh
Pectineus	Found on the inner side of the thigh	Adducts and flexes the femur
Tensor fasciae latae	A flat muscle found along the upper lateral surface of the thigh	Flexes, abducts, and medially rotates the thigh
Rectus femoris	Anterior thigh	Flexes thigh and extends the lower leg
Sartorius (Tailor's muscle)	A long, straplike muscle that runs diagonally across the anterior and medial surface of the thigh	Flexes and rotates the thigh and leg
Gracilis	A long, thin muscle on the medial surface of the thigh	Adducts and flexes the thigh, rotates thigh medially, and flexes leg at knee
Gastrocnemius	Calf muscle	Points toes and flexes the lower leg
Soleus	A broad flat muscle found beneath the gastrocnemius	Extends foot
Peroneus longus	A superficial muscle found on the lateral side of the leg	Extends and everts the foot and supports arches

muscular contraction. The effects of training regarding muscle efficiency are improved coordination of all muscles, improvement of the respiratory and circulatory systems, elimination or reduction of excess fat, and improved joint movement. (See Table 4–8.)

Physiotherapy

Physiotherapy is the treatment of disease and injury by physical means, using light, heat, cold, water, electricity, massage, and exercise.

> *The correct type of massage is essential when providing the proper physiotherapy or a general sense of well-being to the client. Use Figure 4–8 to become familiar with the skeletal muscles that may be involved in the performance of massage services in the beauty care industry.*

In order for the trained professional to perform a full-body massage, a full massage service area, complete with supplies, equipment, and a record-keeping system, is essential. The following is a checklist of the supplies and equipment that are generally needed.

Massage room equipment

Supply and linen cabinets	Chairs
Massage tables	Stool
Bolsters and pillows	Bolster and pillow covers
Sheets	Blankets
Indirect lighting	

Changing room equipment

Hangers (clothing)	Chair or bench
Small table	

Exercise equipment

Stretching bars	Weight lifts
Stationary bicycle	

Supply cabinet

Towels	Sheets
Pillows and cases	Bolsters and covers
Blankets or coverlets	Disposable paper slippers
Tape measure	Room measure
Mouth thermometer	Facial cosmetics
Talcum powder	Massage creams, oils
Moist hot packs	Cold packs
Cotton for facial cleansing	Facial tissues
Cotton-tipped swabs	Sterilizing agent
Table salt for salt glows	Record cards
Watch with second hand	Robes or kimonos
Alcohol or other sterilizing agents	Analgesic oil for sore or stiff muscles

Physical therapy equipment

Standard weight chart	Anatomical wall chart
Bathroom scales	Standard height chart
Heat lamp	Massage table
Shower room	Massage vibrator
Bath cabinet	Shampoo slab
Bathtub	Foot basin
Electrical apparatus	Wall plate

Preparing the client for the massage should include the following steps: initial client consultation; taking the pulse and temperature of the client; filling out the record, consultation, and information forms; and draping the client. (Draping is performed for the purposes of maintaining client comfort, modesty, and warmth.)

Table 4–8   Skeletal Muscles Involved in Massage

NAME OF SKELETAL MUSCLE	LOCATION
Sternocleiodomastoid	Side of the neck
Trapezius	Back of the neck and upper back
Latissimus dorsi	Lower back
Pectoralis major	Chest
Serratus anterior	Lateral ribs
External oblique	Anterior and lateral abdomen
Deltoid	Shoulder
Biceps brachii	Anterior aspect of arm
Triceps brachii	Posterior aspect of arm
Brachioradialis	Anterior and proximal forearm
Gluteus maximus	Buttock
Tensor fascia latae	Lateral and Proximal Thigh
Sartorius	Anterior thigh
Quadriceps femoris group (rectus femoris, vastus lateralis, vastus medialis, vastus intermedius)	Anterior thigh
Hamstring group (biceps, femoris, semitendinosus, semimembranosus)	Posterior thigh
Gracilis	Medial thigh
Tibialis anterior	Anterior leg
Gastrocnemius	Posterior leg
Soleus	Posterior (Deep) leg
Peroneus longus	Lateral leg

There are any number of massage manipulation combinations that can be tailored to the needs of a client. The following classic movements have originated from Swedish massage techniques. The practitioner must understand which movements fall into which category.

Most massage treatments combine one or more of these movements, as divided into the seven major categories:

Classification of Massage Movements

1. Touch
    a. Superficial
    b. Deep
2. Effleurage or stroking movements.
    a. Superficial
        i. Feathering
        ii. Applying oil
    b. Deep
        i. Over large surfaces
        ii. Over heavier muscles
3. Petrissage movements
    a. Kneading
    b. Pulling
4. Fiction (these are considered to be compression movements).
    a. Wringing
    b. Rolling
    c. Chucking
    d. Compression
    e. Circular friction
    f. Transverse or cross-fiber friction
5. Percussion movements
    a. Tapping (tapotement)
    b. Slapping
    c. Cupping
    d. Hacking
    e. Beating
6. Vibration
    a. Manual
    b. Mechanical
7. Joint movements
    a. Passive
    b. Active
        i. Active assistive
        ii. Passive resistive

Each manipulation is applied in a specific way for a specific purpose. The practitioner must regulate the intensity of the pressure, the direction of movement. and the duration of each type of manipulation.

NOTE: Muscular tissues can be stimulated by any of the following:

1. Chemicals—certain acids and salts.
2. Massage—hand massage and appliances, such as vibrators.
3. Electric current—high-frequency.
4. Light rays—infrared rays.
5. Heat rays—heating lamps and masks.
6. Moist heat—steamers or warm steam towels.
7. Nerve impulses—through the nervous system.

> *When performing facial services the professional will be concerned with the voluntary muscles of the head, face, and neck. It is essential to know where these muscles are located and what movements they control. (Refer to Figure 4–1.)*

Massage movements over small areas, such as the face, are performed with the fingertips and palms. Generally, the massage movement is directed from the insertion to the origin of the muscles in order to avoid damage to delicate muscular tissues.

> **NOTE:** The origin of a muscle is the more fixed attachment, as with muscles attached to bones or to some other muscle (see no. 5 in Figure 4–1). The insertion of a muscle is the more movable attachment, as with muscles attached to a movable muscle, to a movable bone, or the skin (see muscle no. 8 in Figure 4–1).

For the correct position for stroking, the fingers should be slightly curved with the cushions of the fingertips touching the skin. (Avoid touching the skin with the tips of the nails.) Stroking has a soothing effect. (Figure 4–2.)

The correct position for palmar stroking is to keep the wrist and fingers flexible, while curving the fingers to conform to the shape of the area being massaged. (See Figures 4–3 and 4–4.)

The kneading move requires that the skin be grasped gently between the thumb and the forefinger. As the tissues are lifted from their underlying structures, they are squeezed, rolled, or pinched with a gentle but firm pressure. A smooth, rhythmic movement should be used. Kneading movements give deeper stimulation, improve circulation, and help empty the oil ducts. (See Figure 4–5.)

Friction is a movement that requires light pressure on the skin while it is moved over the underlying structures. Friction provides a marked benefit to the circulation and glandular activity of the skin. (See Figure 4–6.)

Percussion is performed through tapping, slapping, or hacking movements. In tapping, the fingertips are brought down against the skin in rapid succession, with enough coordination to create an even force over the area being treated. This is the most stimulating form of massage and should be performed with extreme care. (See Figure 4–7 on page 84.)

Slapping movements require flexible wrists to permit the palms to come in contact with the skin in very light, firm, and rapid movements, in which one hand follows the other in a rhythmic manner. When used in facial massage, care must be taken to apply only gentle movements. (See Figure 4–8 on page 84.)

Vibration or shaking movements are accomplished by making rapid muscular contractions in the arms while pressing the fingertips firmly on the point of application. Because this is a highly stimulating movement, it should be used sparingly and should never exceed a few seconds' duration on any one spot. (See Figure 4–9 on page 84.)

Basic Scalp Massage

The basic scalp massage is performed for the purpose of relaxation and should not be confused with the full scalp treatments and massage that are given by professional cosmetologists and barber-stylists.

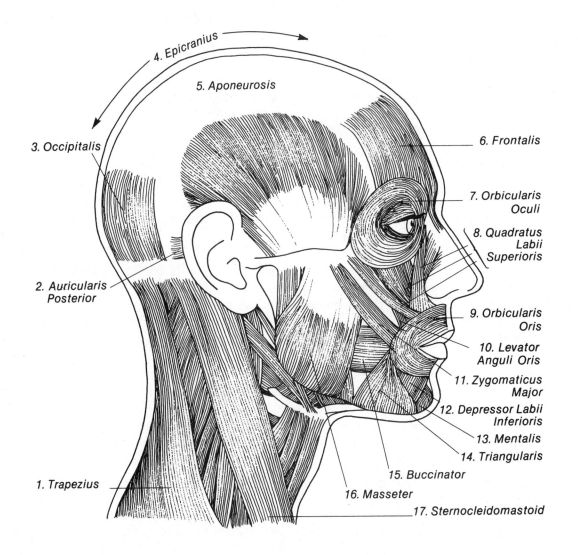

4. Epicranius

5. Aponeurosis

3. Occipitalis

6. Frontalis

7. Orbicularis
   Oculi

8. Quadratus
   Labii
   Superioris

2. Auricularis
   Posterior

9. Orbicularis
   Oris

10. Levator
    Anguli Oris

11. Zygomaticus
    Major

12. Depressor Labii
    Inferioris

13. Mentalis

14. Triangularis

1. Trapezius

15. Buccinator

16. Masseter

17. Sternocleidomastoid

Figure 4-1   Muscles of the head, face, and neck

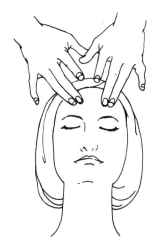

Figure 4–2 Effleurage

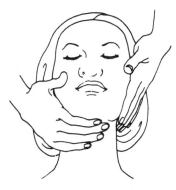

Figure 4–3 Digital and palmar stroking of the face

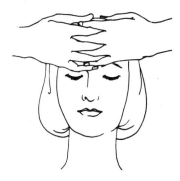

Figure 4–4 The correct position for palmar stroking

When performing the basic scalp massage, apply firm pressure on upward strokes as illustrated in the "Scalp Massage Procedure." (See Figure 4–10.) Firm rotary movements are given to loosen scalp tissues, which tends to improve the health of the hair and scalp by increasing the circulation of blood to the scalp and hair papillae. Use steady, slow manipulations and take care not to pull the hair in any way.

Musculoskeletal Disorders

Injury and disease may interfere with the coordination and functions of muscles. Rehabilitation in the form of therapeutic exercise is the retraining of injured or unused muscles. Muscle atrophy (shrinkage and lost muscle strength) can occur due to infrequently used muscles, prolonged bedrest, or the immobilization of a limb.

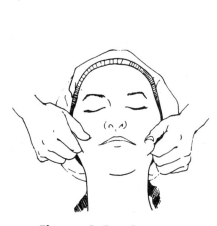

Figure 4–5 Petrissage

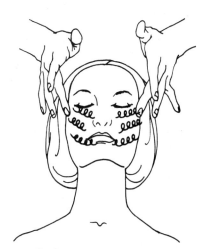

Figure 4–6 Friction

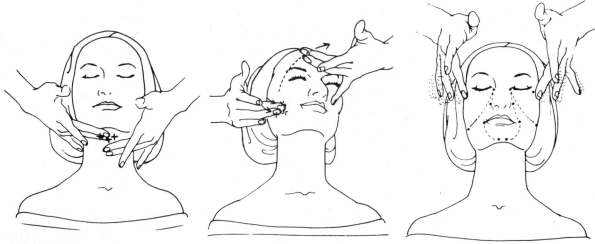

Figure 4-7   Percussion or tapotement

Figure 4-8   Slapping movements

Figure 4-9   Vibration or shaking movements

Muscle atrophy can be minimized by direct electrical stimulation, massage, or special exercise.

There are several musculoskeletal disorders that can affect the professional especially frequently. These include the following conditions:

Flatfeet (as previously discussed) are the result of the downward pressure of the body weight on the foot, which flattens the arches due to a weakening of the leg muscles. Muscle strength may be increased by exercise, massage, and electrical stimulation.

Muscle hypertrophy results from overworking or overexercising, whereby the muscle enlarges and becomes stronger.

Muscle fatigue may occur from the temporary overuse of muscles. An athletic massage prior to a workout can help prevent muscle injury and fatigue.

A stiff neck, especially in the beauty care field, may be due to an inflammation (caused by overuse of the muscle) of the trapezius muscle. Regular exercise is an effective preventative and massage is an excellent treatment for this condition.

Muscle spasms (sudden and violent contractions) may be caused by the sudden overworking of a muscle or by poor circulation to the localized area.

Myalgia is muscular pain.

Professionals in the beauty care industry can attest to the myriad tensions, pressures, and strains that occur during the average workday. The legs, lower back, shoulder, and neck areas appear to be the most affected by the daily twisting, bending, arm extensions, and standing that are so much a part of the profession. The best preventative measures include regular exercise, good nutrition, practicing good posture, and receiving regular massage.

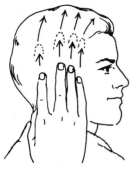

1. Place the fingertips of each hand at the hairline on each side of the client's head, pointing the hands upward. Slide the fingers firmly upward spreading the fingertips. Continue until the fingers meet at the center or top of the scalp. Repeat three or four times.

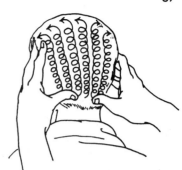

2. Place the fingers of each hand on either side of the client's head behind the ears. Use the thumbs to massage from behind the ears toward the crown. Repeat four or five times. Move your fingers until both thumbs meet at the hairline at the back of the client's neck. Rotate your thumbs upward towards the crown.

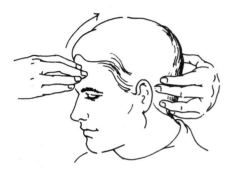

3. Step to the right side of the client. Place the left hand at the back of the head. Place the thumb and fingers of the right hand over the forehead, just above the eyebrows. With the cushion tips of the right hand, thumb and fingers, massage slowly and firmly in an upward direction toward the crown while keeping the left hand in a fixed position at the back of the head. Repeat four or five times.

4. Step to the back of the client. a) Place the hands on each side of the head, at the front hairline. Rotate the fingertips three times. On the fourth rotation, apply a quick, upward twist, firm enough to move the scalp. b) Continue this movement on the sides and tip of the scalp. Repeat three or four times.

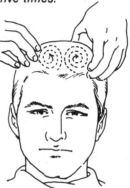

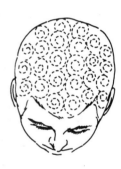

a

b

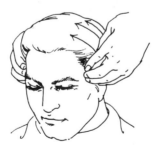

5. Place the fingers (of each hand) below the back of each ear. Rotate the fingers upward from behind the ears to the crown. Repeat three or four times. Move the fingers toward the back of the head, and repeat the movement with both hands. Apply rotary movements in an upward direction toward the crown.

6. Place both hands at the sides of the client's head. Keep the fingers close together, and hold the index fingers at hairline above the ears. Firmly move both hands directly upward to the top of the head. Repeat four times. Move the hands to above the ears and repeat the movement. Move hands again to back of the ears and repeat the movement.

Figure 4–10   The scalp massage procedure

The Effects of Massage

Massage stimulates and tones muscles, helps to relieve soreness and stiffness in muscles and joints, strengthens connective tissues, aids in relaxation, relieves fatigue, provides relief of muscle spasms, and increases circulation.

As beneficial as massage may be for most people, there are certain conditions that make massage unadvisable. The following list provides the name and a brief summary of these conditions:

Abnormal body temperature of over 99.4 degrees Fahrenheit generally indicates that the body is trying to isolate and eliminate an invading pathogen (disease-causing bacteria). Massage may work against the body's defense mechanisms.

Individuals with acute infectious diseases such as typhoid, diphtheria, influenza, and severe colds should avoid massage.

Inflammation of a particular body area may be further irritated or intensified by massage—especially the penetrating types.

Varicose veins is a condition in which the veins break down because of back pressure in the circulatory system, usually caused by pregnancy or long periods of standing. This excessive back pressure causes veins to stretch to the extent that the small valves within the veins, which normally allow blood to move only in one direction, collapse and lose the ability to stop the backward flow of blood. If the flow of blood becomes obstructed, clotting may occur. Any deep massage in these areas may set a blood clot loose in the general circulation and cause a serious problem.

Inflammation of a vein accompanied by pain is called phlebitis. Again, if a blood clot forms and a piece of it floats in the blood (an embolus), it has the potential to reach the lungs, causing death; the brain, causing a stroke; or the heart, causing cardiac arrest.

Edema is another circulatory abnormality that is caused by an excess accumulation of fluid in tissue spaces. The presence of edema can be determined by pressing a finger into the area. If an indentation remains after the finger is removed, edema is present.

High blood pressure means pressure of the blood against the walls of the arteries. Because hypertension is a factor of high blood pressure, soothing massage may be of some benefit. Stimulating or deep pressure massage should be avoided, however.

Cancer can become widespread through the lymphatic system, and because massage tends to increase lymph flow, massage is rarely recommended. An exception may be when the massage is limited to simple touch and reflex therapy to provide client comfort and all circulatory types of massage are avoided.

In cases of intoxication, massage is not recommended because it can spread toxins and overstress the liver.

Skin problems usually only affect a given area of the face or body; therefore, massage on unaffected areas is permissible. Massage is never given when a condition is of a contagious nature, however.

Elderly people with a frail nature may have sensitive skin and fragile bones. Gentle massage can be therapeutic and beneficial, but deep pressure should be avoided.

Massage during pregnancy can be beneficial if performed correctly and if client positioning and comfort are taken into consideration. The massage should always be soothing and relaxing, with no heavy deep-tissue or percussion massage being performed.

NOTE: Therapeutic massage is a science in its own right and requires in-depth instruction and practice to perform correctly. The above condition summaries provide the reader with a mere glimpse of the many considerations and technical knowledge required in the performance of therapeutic massage. The level of professional training required to perform massage therapy should be respected and adhered to. Do not attempt any deep or penetrating massage techniques without the proper training.

NOTE: Generally speaking, highly active muscle tissue creates heat that can raise the body's temperature. To counter this effect, blood circulates more quickly through the tissue to diffuse the heat, which is eventually excreted through the skin.

4 Review

Fill in the Blank

1. The ability to move is made possible by the _____ of muscles.

2. Muscle tissue comprises about _____ the total body weight.

3. Muscle provides the following functions: allows the body and individual parts to _____; helps to keep the body _____ and _____; produces _____; participates in the movement of _____; and gives the body _____.

4. The three principle types of muscle are the _____, or striated; _____, or spindle-shaped; and _____ or nonstriated.

5–7. Identify the following muscle types as being voluntary or involuntary.

5. _____ Skeletal

6. _____ Smooth

7. _____ Cardiac

8. The three characteristics that muscles have in common are _____, _____ _____, and _____.

9. Muscles are attached to bones by _____.

10. The _____ of the muscle is attached to a fixed structure that moves least during muscle contraction.

11. The _____ is attached to the movable end and moves the most during a muscle contraction.

12. The _____ is the central area of the muscle.

13. The muscles of the body are arranged in _____.

14. When one muscle produces movement in a single direction, the other muscles does so in the _____ direction.

15. Muscle fatigue is caused by an accumulation of _____ in the muscles.

16. _____ is a condition of a muscle in which it is always slightly contracted and ready to pull.

17. The muscles of the head control _____ and the act of _____ .

18. The muscles of the neck move the head through _____ , _____ , and _____ movements.

19. The muscles of the _____ help move the shoulders, arms, forearms, wrists, hands, and fingers.

20. The muscles of the _____ control breathing and the movements of the abdomen and the pelvis.

21. The muscles of the _____ assist in the movement of the thighs, legs, ankles, feet, and toes.

22. Exercise will alter the _____ , and _____ of a muscle.

23. Physiotherapy is the treatment of disease and injury by _____ means.

24. Physiotherapy may be achieved through the use of _____ , _____ , _____ , _____ , _____ , _____ , and _____ .

25. _____ may be stimulated by chemicals, massage, electric current, light rays, heat rays, moist heat, or nerve impulses.

26. _____ exercise is the retraining of injured or unused muscles.

27. Five musculoskeletal disorders with which the professional may come in contact or experience are: _____ and _____ _____ .

28. Preventative measures for the professional include _____ _____ and _____ .

29. _____ can stimulate and tone muscles, strengthen connective tissue, aid in relaxation, increase circulation and relieve soreness, fatigue and muscle spasms.

30–36. Massage is unadvisable when:

30. _____ .

31. _____ .

32. _____ .

33. _____ .

34. _____ .

35. _____ .

36. _____ .

37. _____ massage should be avoided on elderly people of a fragile nature.

38. Massage during pregnancy should always be of a _____ and _____ nature.

39. There are _____ basic steps to a scalp massage.

Matching

40–44. Match the following massage movements with their definition.

40. _____
41. _____
42. _____
43. _____
44. _____

Kneading	Effleurage
Shaking movement	Friction
Stroking	Percussion
Rubbing	Petrissage
Tapping	Vibration

<table>
<tr><td>

5

</td><td>

Transport of Blood and Oxygen

</td></tr>
</table>

Blood is transported throughout the body through a system of blood vessels known as a closed circulatory system. This is the largest organ of the body. (See Figure 5–1.)

Functions of Blood

The blood helps the body maintain a stable internal environment, which is essential to the proper carrying out of the body's activities.

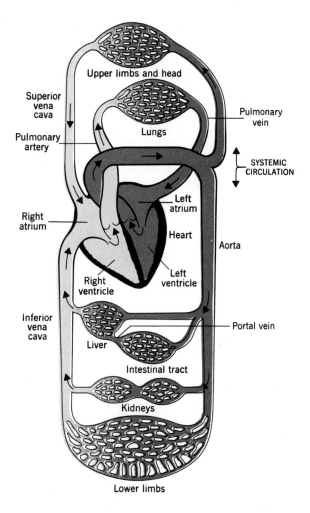

Figure 5–1   The circulatory system

Blood is a liquid tissue composed of **plasma** (the fluid component) and **blood cells** (the solid component). Blood cells include red blood cells, white blood cells, and platelets. Red blood cells carry oxygen to the cells for oxidation and carbon dioxide away for excretion. White blood cells protect against disease by engulfing and digesting bacteria and foreign matter that have invaded the body. Platelets assist in the clotting action of blood when bleeding occurs.

Plasma suspends blood cells, transports them throughout the body, bring nutrients to the cells, and carries away metabolic waste products to the excretory organs. Within the excretory organs, the waste products are converted into chemical compounds called hormones, which are then secreted into the plasma. The plasma circulates the hormones to various parts of the body, where they help to regulate bodily functions.

Another essential function of blood is that it helps the body maintain its water content and body temperature. (Excessive body temperature can disrupt chemical reactions in the cells.) Finally, blood helps maintain the body's internal acid balance by creating chemicals in the bloodstream known as bicarbonates and phosphates which neutralize small amounts of acids or alkalis. (See Table 5–1.)

Blood does not leave the blood vessels to flow through the tissues but remains inside as it is transported throughout the body, to form a closed circuit of blood. The

FUNCTION	EFFECT ON BODY
Nutritive	Transporting nutrient molecules (glucose, amino acids, fatty acids, and glycerol) from the small intestine or storage sites to the tissues
Respiratory	Transporting oxygen from the lungs to the tissues and carbon dioxide from the tissues to the lungs
Excretory	Transporting waste products (lactic acid, urea, and creatinine) from the cells to the excretory organs
Regulatory	Transporting hormones and other chemical substances that control the proper functioning of many organs
	Circulating excess heat to the body surfaces and to the lungs, through which it is lost (controls body temperature)
	Maintains water balance and a constant environment for tissue cells
Protective	Circulating antibodies and defensive cells throughout the body to combat infection and disease

Table 5–1   Summary of the Various Functions of Blood

blood circuit contains arteries and small artery branches, veins, venules (small veins), and capillaries. Blood is pumped through the blood vessels by the action of the heart.

The circulatory system also includes the lymphatic system. This consists of lymph and tissue fluid originating from the blood and lymphatic vessels, which return the lymph to the blood.

Major Blood Circuits

With the exception of pulmonary circulation, the blood leaves the heart through the arteries and returns by the veins, creating two circulation routes:

1. The general or systemic circulation carries blood throughout the body. (See Figure 5–2.)
2. The pulmonary circulation carries blood from the heart to the lungs and back again. (See Table 5–2.)

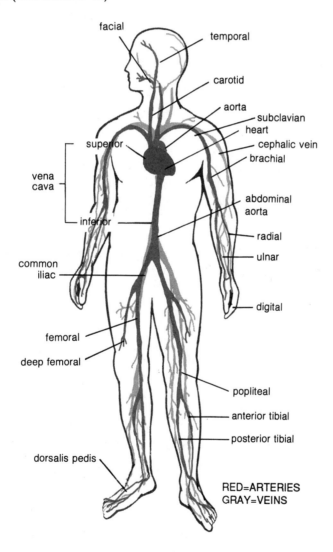

Figure 5–2   General or systemic circulation

ORGANS	BLOOD LOSES	BLOOD GAINS
Digestive glands	Raw materials needed to make digestive juices and enzymes	Carbon dioxide
Kidneys	Water, urea, and mineral salts	Carbon dioxide
Liver	Excess glucose, amino acids, and worn-out red blood cells	Released glucose, urea, and plasma proteins
Lungs	Carbon dioxide and water	Oxygen
Muscles	Glucose and oxygen	Lactic acid and carbon dioxide
Small intestinal villi	Oxygen	End products of digestion (glucose and amino acids)

Table 5-2 Changes in the composition of the Blood

The Heart

The heart is a tough, simply constructed muscle about the size of a closed fist, measuring approximately 5 inches long and 3 1/2 inches wide, and weighing less than a pound (12–13 ounces). Its obvious purpose is to circulate life-sustaining blood throughout the body. The heart is located within the thoracic cavity, between the lungs, behind the sternum and above the diaphragm. The heart's conical tip lies on the diaphragm and points to the left of the body, which can be where the heartbeat is most easily felt and heard.

> **NOTE:** The life-saving technique known as cardiopulmonary resuscitation (CPR) should be performed only by those trained in the technique.

Structure of the Heart

The heart is a hollow, muscular, double pump that can circulate approximately 75 gallons of blood per hour. Surrounding the heart is the pericardium, a double layer of fibrous tissue that contains a lubricating fluid (pericardial fluid) between the two layers.

Cardiac muscle tissue (myocardium) makes up the wall of the heart, with an inner lining of smooth tissue called the endocardium, which covers the heart valves and lines the blood vessel to provide smooth transit for the flowing blood.

The heart is separated into right and left halves by the septum, which completely separates the blood in each side as well. The right side of the heart carries only deoxygenated blood, and the left side, only oxygenated blood. (See Figure 5–3.)

Each half is divided into two parts, creating four chambers in all. The two upper chambers are referred to as the right atrium and the left atrium (also known as auricles). The lower chambers are the right ventricle and the left ventricle.

The atrioventricular valves and the semilunar valves permit the blood to flow in only one direction, prohibiting it from flowing backward into the chambers.

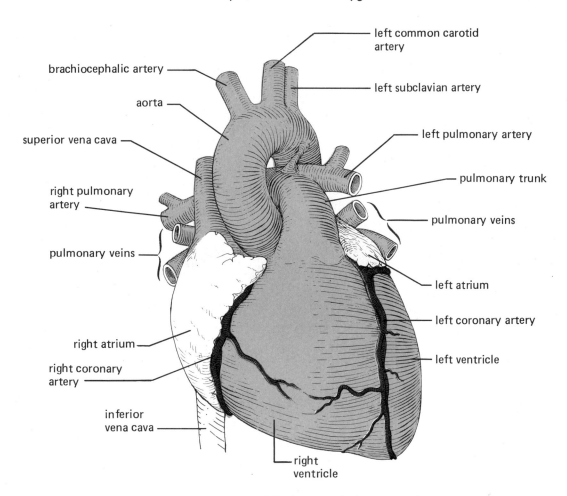

Figure 5-3   Anterior view of the heart with the pericardium removed

The tricuspid valve allows blood flow from the right atrium into the right ventricle, but not in the opposite direction.

The mitral bicuspid valve allows blood flow from the left atrium to the left ventricle.

The pulmonary semilunar valve lets blood travel from the right ventricle into the pulmonary artery and then into the lungs.

The aortic semilunar valve permits the blood to pass from the left ventricle into the aorta. (See Figure 5–4.)

The heartbeat generates in the heart muscle itself, where the myocardium contracts rhythmically, causing it to perform as a pump. The control of heart muscle contractions is found within a group of conducting cells, known as the sinoatrial (S-A) node, which send out electrical impulses that make the atria contact simultaneously. This causes downward blood flow from the upper atrial chamber to the atrioventricular openings. Eventually, the electrical impulse will reach the atrioventricular (A-V) node—another conducting cell group located between the atria and ventricle. The electrical impulse is then carried to conducting fibers in the septum, which branch out until they reach the heart's apex.

The combined action of the S-A and A-V nodes is instrumental in the cardiac cycle, which is composed of one complete heartbeat involving both atrial and ventricle contractions.

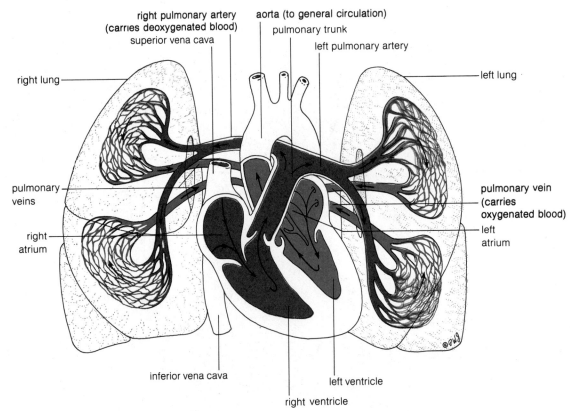

right pulmonary artery
(carries deoxygenated blood)
superior vena cava

aorta (to general circulation)
pulmonary trunk
left pulmonary artery

right lung

left lung

pulmonary
veins

pulmonary vein
(carries
oxygenated blood)

right
atrium

left
atrium

inferior vena cava

left ventricle

right ventricle

Figure 5-4   Pulmonary circulation

Function and Path of General Circulation

There are four main functions of the general circulation: it circulates nutrients, oxygen, water, and secretions to tissues and then back to the heart; it carries carbon dioxide and other dissolved wastes away from tissues; it helps equalize body temperature; and it aids in protecting the body from pathogenic bacteria.

The blood can return to the heart from the arms or the legs. Blood that flows from the upper part of the body (head, neck, and arms) returns to the right side of the heart through the superior vena cava, one of the two largest veins in the body.

Blood from the lower part of the body (legs and trunk) enters the heart through the inferior vena cava, the other of the two largest veins. Blood enters the right atrium from both these veins, which then contract, forcing the blood through the tricuspid valve into the right ventricle. This chamber contains deoxygenated blood, which contains little oxygen and a good deal of carbon dioxide.

The right ventricle contracts to push the deoxygenated blood through the pulmonary semilunar valve into the pulmonary trunk, where it branches into the right and left pulmonary arteries, bringing deoxygenated blood to the right and left lungs, respectively. Once in the lungs, gaseous exchange takes place: carbon dioxide leaves the red blood cells and is discharged, to be excreted from the lungs. Oxygen combines with hemoglobin in the red blood cells, where it then travels into small veins and venules. The right pulmonary veins carry oxygenated blood from the right lung to the heart and into the left atrium. From the left lung, blood enters the left atrium through the two left pulmonary veins. The left atrium contacts, sending blood through the mitral valve into the left ventricle, which acts as a pump for the newly oxygenated blood. When the left ventricle contracts, it sends oxygenated blood through the aorta seilunar valve and then into the aorta.

The aorta is the largest artery in the body and forms an arch, consisting of three branches: the brachycephalic, the left common carotid, and the left subclavian arteries. These ascending aorta arteries and their branches carry blood to the arms, neck, and head.

The descending aorta arteries carry oxygenated blood throughout the body. The first branch, the coronary artery, carries blood to the heart's muscular wall. Additional branches of the descending aorta reach the stomach, intestines, liver, pancreas, reproductive organs, legs, and so forth. Each of these arteries subdivides into smaller arteries, then into arterioles, and finally into capillaries embedded in the tissues. This is the juncture where hormones, nutrients, oxygen, and other materials are transferred from the blood into the tissues. (See Figure 5–5.)

In summary, the pulmonary circulation carries blood from the heart to the lungs and back to the heart again. The pulmonary trunk carries deoxygenated blood, which is exchanged for a new oxygen supply in the lungs. Pulmonary circulation starts its circuit by leaving the right ventricle of the heart (through the pulmonary trunk), carrying deoxygenated blood into a right pulmonary artery traveling to the right lung and into a left pulmonary artery into the left lung. The two arteries eventually branch out into capillaries inside the lungs, where the exchange of carbon dioxide and oxygen take place. The newly oxygenated blood returns to the heart through the right and left pulmonary veins, where it enters the left atrium of the heart. It is now ready to complete the circuit throughout the body via the general circulation.

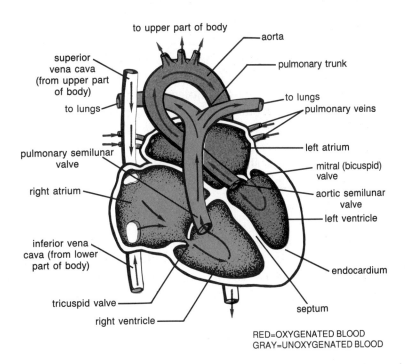

Figure 5–5 Schematic of pulmonary circulation

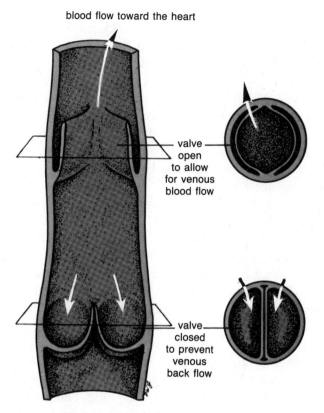

blood flow toward the heart

valve
open
to allow
for venous
blood flow

valve
closed
to prevent
venous
back flow

Figure 5–6   Valves in the vein

NOTE: Generally, arteries carry oxygenated blood away from the heart to the capillaries. The only exception is the pulmonary artery system, which carries deoxygenated blood from the heart to the lungs. Veins, on the other hand, carry deoxygenated blood away from the capillaries to the heart in venules (small veins). Capillaries are an endothelial cell layer that connects the arterioles with venules, allowing for the selective permeability of other cells and substances. Nutrient molecules and oxygen can pass out of the capillaries and into surrounding tissues, and metabolic wastes can be passed back into the bloodstream for proper excretion. Capillaries also serve the function of allowing white blood cells to leave the bloodstream and enter tissue spaces to assist in the destruction of invading bacteria. (See Figure 5–6.)

The structure of the veins should be understood by the professional for the purpose of preventing or coping with a varicose vein condition on either a personal or client service basis.

Veins are less elastic, thinner-walled, and less muscular than arteries. The thinner wall of the vein can collapse easily when it is not filled with blood. Additionally, veins have intermittent valves along their length which allow the blood to flow in only one direction, towards the heart, and prevent the backflow of blood toward the capillaries.

Varicose veins are enlarged, swollen veins (occurring most often in the legs) which result from the slowing up of blood flow back to the heart due to the breakdown in the valves. When the valves do not function properly, blood accumulates and backs up, causing distention and inelasticity of the vein walls.

One of the most significant contributing factors to the formation of varicose veins is lack of circulation brought on by one or more of the following considerations: prolonged periods of standing or sitting, crossing the legs while sitting, heredity, lack of exercise, being overweight or pregnant, and advancing age.

It should be readily apparent to the professional that the physical demands of the beauty care profession may increase the risk of developing varicose veins, especially while working during the advanced stages of pregnancy. Care should be taken to wear quality support hose and to take occasional breaks while on the job, elevating the legs if possible. Proper nutrition, exercise, and certain herbal or vitamin supplements such as N, N-Dimethylglycine (for improved cell oxygen utilization), Vitamin C (for the reduction of blood-clotting tendencies), and Butcher's Broom (good for all types of circulatory disorders and the relief of inflammation), may prove beneficial for preventative and corrective measures.

NOTE: The effects of massage in relation to varicose veins is discussed in Chapter 5, The "Muscular System"

Blood Pressure

As the heart pumps blood into the arteries, the surge of blood filling the vessels creates pressure against the arterial walls. Systolic blood pressure is the pressure at the moment of the heart muscle's contraction, which is caused by the rush of blood that follows ventricle contractions. It refers to the pressure exerted by the blood while the heart is pumping, indicating the highest level of blood pressure. When the ventricles of the heart muscle are relaxed and at rest between beats, the force of the blood is lessened. This is known as diastolic pressure.

The blood pressure–measuring device is called a sphygmomanometer and measures readings in a ratio of the systolic blood pressure to the diastolic blood pressure. The mercury within the tube of the sphygmomanometer rises under the pressure exerted by the blood. Normal blood pressure readings may vary from 110/70 to 140/90, but 120/80 is the most accepted normal reading. Readings of 140/90 to 160/90 may indicate marginal hypertension, while any reading over 180/115 indicates a severe condition.

High blood pressure is a common, but nonetheless potentially dangerous, condition that can often lead to heart attacks and strokes. High blood pressure can also be a factor in kidney and thyroid disorders, diabetes, and obesity. Symptoms of hypertension may include sweating, dizziness, headache, rapid pulse, shortness of breath, and vision irregularities. Blood pressure should be checked on a regular basis, especially for individuals in high-risk groups.

There are several services offered by professionals, especially in full-service shops and salons, that may incur risk to the client with high blood pressure. These include facials (most notably, those performed with steam towels), full body massages, body wraps, tanning booths, and the like. If a client has a history of high blood pressure, do not perform these services. If you are unsure about a client's health status and wish to make a more informed determination about the possible risk factors, take the client's pulse, temperature, and blood pressure as part of the client consultation and preparation procedure.

NOTE: Check with your state board concerning any possible restriction or certificate training that may be required in order to perform these services on the general public.

Pulse

A pulse is an alternating expansion and contraction of the artery as blood flows through it. The following is a list of six locations on the body where the pulse may conveniently be felt: the brachial artery—located at the crook of the elbow; the common carotid artery—found in the neck along the sternocleidomastoid muscle; the dorsalis pedis artery—on the anterior surface of the foot, below the ankle joint; the facial artery—located at the lower edge of the mandible, aligned with the corner of the mouth, the radial artery—at the wrist, on the posterior surface of the radius; and the temporal artery—found slightly above the outer edge of the eye. The pulse rate of an adult female is 80 beats per minute; it is 78 beats per minute for the adult male.

The Blood

As previously discussed, the blood is a transporting fluid of the body that carries nutrients from the digestive tract to the cells, oxygen from the lungs to the cells, waste products from the cells to various organs for excretion, and hormones from secreting cells to other part of the body. Blood also aids in heat distribution, helps regulate the acid-base balance, and protects against infection.

The liquid portion of blood is called plasma and contains various types of dissolved chemicals and several different types of blood cells.

Blood Plasma

Plasma is a straw-colored liquid making up approximately 55 percent of the blood volume and containing the following substances: water—about 92 percent of the total volume of plasma, it is maintained by the kidneys and by water intake and output; and blood protein—a protein found in red blood cells known as hemoglobin.

Plasma proteins include fibrinogen, necessary for blood clotting; serum albumin, which helps maintain osmotic pressure and volume and provides the "pulse pressure" needed to hold and pull water from tissue fluid back into the blood vessels; serum globulin, which is formed in the liver and lymphatic system; gamma globulin, which helps to synthesize antibodies; and prothrombin, which also helps blood to coagulate.

Nutrients in molecular form are absorbed, while glucose, fatty acids, cholesterol, and amino acids are dissolved in the blood plasma.

Mineral salts (electrolytes) act as chemical buffers in helping to maintain the acid-base balance of the blood.

Hormones, vitamins and enzymes help the body to control its chemical reactions.

Metabolic waste products are formed by the chemical reactions occurring to maintain homeostasis.

Red Blood Cells

Red blood cells, or **erythrocytes (eh-RITH-rho-seyets)**, contain the red pigment hemoglobin, which is composed of protein and iron. Hemoglobin is vital to the function of the red blood cell as it helps transport oxygen to the tissues and carbon dioxide away from them. Erythropoiesis is the synthesis of red blood cells, which occurs in the red bone marrow of all bones until adolescence.

White Blood Cells

White blood cells, or **leukocytes (LOO-koh-seyets)**, are synthesized in red bone marrow and in lymphatic tissue. Leukocytes help protect the body against infection and injury by surrounding and digesting or destroying bacteria, by the synthesis of antibody molecules, by "cleaning up" cellular remains at inflammation sites, and by walling off infected areas. (See Figure 5–7.)

Inflammation. Inflammation occurs when living tissue is damaged by chemical or physical trauma or through the invasion of pathogenic bacteria. Characteristic symptoms of inflammation include redness, localized heat, swelling, and pain. In most inflammations, a combination forms of dead tissue, dead and living bacteria, dead leukocytes and blood plasma (called pus). If the damaged area is below the epidermis, an abscess (pus-filled cavity) will form. If the damaged area is on the skin, it is called an ulcer.

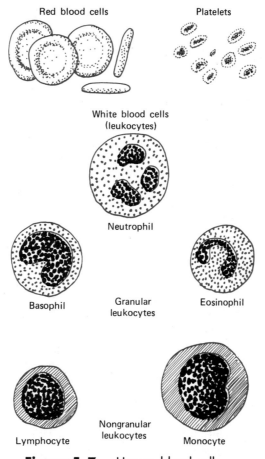

Figure 5–7   Human blood cells

Blood Platelets

Blood platelets (**thrombocytes**) are the smallest solid components of blood and function in the initial blood-clotting process by producing adhesive structures that stick to collegen fibers in a wound to stop the bleeding. Eventually, the blood-clotting process follows to "harden" the platelet plug and closes the wound. Blood coagulation is dependent on the blood platelets which indirectly require vitamin K. Coagulation should occur in from four to six minutes in humans.

Most professionals have had to deal with the occasional nick, cut, or scratch in the performance of services. More often than not, they are the injured party! Shears slip, the client moves unexpectedly, or a razor is mishandled. We are well used to taking care of these minor mishaps. However, when the client is the one to suffer the injury, appropriate first aid measures should be taken. Always inform the client of the accident if he or she is not already aware of it. This is not as unusual as it may sound: due to the extreme sharpness of many of the tools and implements used, the client might not feel the cut or nick immediately. If it appears that a minor cut is not clotting within the average time frame, call a physician or recommend that your client sees his or her own physician as soon as possible.

Blood Types

Blood type is inherited from one's parents and is determined by the presence or absence of a blood protein, called agglutinogen, on the surface of the red blood cell. The four blood types are A, B, AB, and O. Agglutinogens are either A or B and are present individually, as in Type A and Type B blood; jointly, as in the AB blood type; or not at all, as in the O blood type.

Another factor for consideration is the protein in the plasma, known as agglutinin, which is the opposite of the agglutinogens present in that blood type. For example, Type A blood has b agglutinin, Type B has a agglutinin, Type AB has no agglutinin, and Type O possesses both a and b agglutinin. Agglutinins react with the agglutinogens of the same type, causing the red blood cells to cluster together and resulting in congestion in the blood vessels. This, in turn, causes the impediment of the circulation, which will result in death. A person must receive the right type of blood during transfusions to avoid this fatal result.

RH Factor

Human red cells also contain the RH antigen. Antigens are substances that stimulate the formation of antibodies against themselves. If the RH factor is found on the surface of an individual's red blood cells, the blood is RH positive. When the RH antigen is not present, the blood is considered RH negative. Both blood type and RH factor must be taken into consideration for a successful transfusion.

When an RH negative mother is pregnant with an RH positive fetus, the mother's blood can develop anti-RH agglutinins to the fetus's RH agglutinogens. The firstborn child may not suffer any harmful effects; however, subsequent pregnancies will be affected because the mother's accumulated anti-RH agglutinins will cause the baby's red blood cells to cluster. If the condition is left untreated, the baby will usually be born anemic.

The Lymphatic System and Immunity

The lymphatic system can be considered a supplement to the circulatory system and consists of lymph, lymph nodes, lymph vessels, the spleen, the thymus gland, lymphoid tissue, and the tonsils. (See Figure 5–8.)

Lymph is a straw-colored fluid composed of water, lymphocytes, granulocytes, oxygen, digested nutrients, hormones, salts, carbon dioxide, and urea. Lymph acts as an intermediary between the blood in the capillaries and the tissues and carries digested food, oxygen, and hormones to the cells. It also carries metabolic waste products away from the cells and back into the capillaries for excretion.

Lymph vessels accompany and parallel the veins and are located in most of the tissues and organs that have blood vessels.

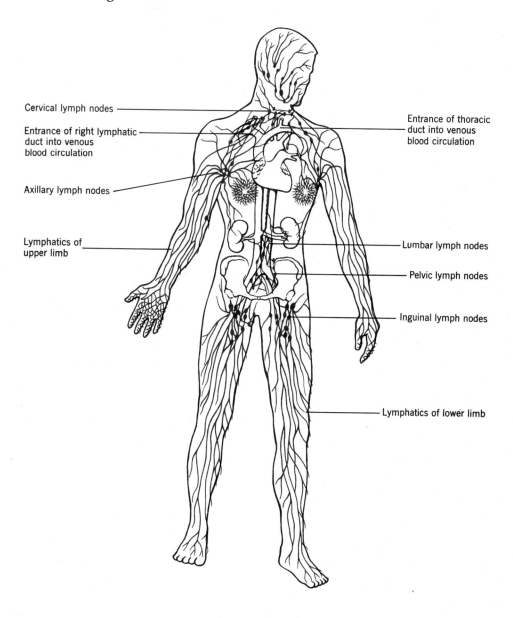

Cervical lymph nodes

Entrance of right lymphatic duct into venous blood circulation

Axillary lymph nodes

Lymphatics of upper limb

Entrance of thoracic duct into venous blood circulation

Lumbar lymph nodes

Pelvic lymph nodes

Inguinal lymph nodes

Lymphatics of lower limb

Figure 5–8   Lymphatic circulation

Lymph nodes are situated either alone or grouped in various places along the lymph vessels throughout the body. Their function is to provide sites for lymphatic production and to serve as a filter for screening out harmful substances from the lymph.

The spleen is a mass of lymphatic tissue that forms lymphocytes and monocytes, filters blood, stores large amounts of red blood cells, forces red blood cells into the circulation when needed, and removes old red blood cells.

The thymus gland is located in the upper anterior part of the thorax, just above the heart. Its function is to produce lymphocytes.

Natural and Acquired Immunities

There are two general types of immunity—natural and acquired. Natural immunity is an inherited, permanent immunity with which we are born. It includes the unbroken skin, cellular secretions (such as mucus and tears), blood phagocytes, and local inflammation.

Acquired immunity is a reaction that occurs as a result of exposure to invaders of the body and is developed over the span of a lifetime. There are two types of acquired immunity: **passive** and **active**. Passive acquired immunity is acquired artificially through the injection of antibodies, which act immediately to provide temporary protection that lasts from three to five weeks. Active acquired immunity is preferable and lasts longer than passive immunity. It is further broken down into two types: natural acquired immunity and artificial acquired immunity. Natural acquired immunity is the result of the body producing antibodies after having had, and recovered from, a particular disease. Artificial acquired immunity is the result of having been inoculated with the appropriate vaccine, antigen, or toxoid.

Immunization is the process of increasing an individual's resistance to a particular infection by artificial means. An antigen is a substance that is injected to stimulate the production of antibodies. An immunoglobulin is a protein that functions specifically as an antibody.

Hypersensitivity

Hypersensitivity occurs when the body's immune system fails to protect itself against foreign material. The antibodies that are formed irritate certain body cells. A hypersensitive or allergic individual is more sensitive to certain allergens than other people. Allergens are antigens, such as grass, pollen, penicillin, and insect stings, that cause allergic responses.

The importance of being able to recognize an allergic reaction cannot be overstressed to the professional. Given the hundreds of chemical products in use by professionals on still more hundreds of clients, its surprising that we aren't witness to more allergic reactions than we usually experience in a lifetime.

"Preventative medicine" is always the best method, when available, and the client consultation is the first step in the prevention of adverse reactions. If a client is receiving chemical services for the first time and no reaction composite is available, be sure to inquire about the client's comfort—is the solution burning, itching, or causing inflammation? Be observant and make notes on the client record card for future reference. Allergies can affect the bronchial membranes, mucous membranes of the respiratory tract, or the skin. The

symptoms of an allergic reaction may include, but are not limited to, difficulty in breathing, dizziness, fainting, headache, swelling, rashes, inflammation, and nausea. If a client should experience an allergic reaction during the course of a service, the professional should be guided by the degree of severity. For instance, if a localized rash appears, simply rinsing with water may alleviate the worst of the problem by removing the offending product; however, in any and all cases where breathing is difficult, call for emergency assistance.

Disorders of the Circulatory System

Disorders of the Heart

Cardiovascular disease is one of the leading causes of death and may be the result of one or more of the following disorders. (Figure 5–9.)

Acute rheumatic heart disease is an infection of the membrane lining of the heart, most often caused by streptococci bacteria, that alters heart tissue and affects the valves, causing heart damage. Any subsequent infections will cause further damage.

Arrhythmia (ay-RITH-mee-ah) is any change from the normal, synchronized rhythm of the heart action.

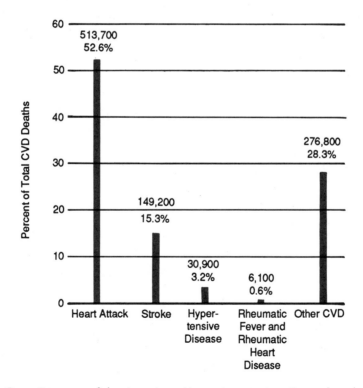

Estimated Deaths Due to Major Cardiovascular Diseases

United States: 1987 Estimate

Figure 5–9   *Courtesy of the American Heart Association. Reproduced with permission.*

Atrial fibrillation is a condition in which the atria are never completely emptied of blood and their walls quiver instead of performing the usual contraction. This is due to weak and irregular nerve impulses which, in turn, cause an irregular wrist pulse and abnormal heart rate.

Congenital heart disease is a condition that is present at birth in which the heart did not develop properly in the uterus.

Endocarditis is another inflammation of the membrane lining. The formation of rough spots in the endocardium may lead to fatal blood clots.

Heart block is the loss of ability of a damaged A-V node (such as blockage in a coronary artery) to carry nerve impulses. The heart block causes the ventricles to contract at a slow, irregular rate. This is usually treated by the implantation of a battery-powered pacemaker, which stimulates the heart electrically to effect the ventricular contractions.

Heart failure is the inability of the heart muscles to beat efficiently and may be caused by high blood pressure or other pathological conditions. Symptoms may include difficult or rapid breathing, the swelling of organs with certain body fluids, lung congestion, and coughing.

Congestive heart failure is similar to heart failure, with the addition of swelling in the lower extremities. Blood backs up into the lung vessels and fluid extend into the air passages.

Angina pectoris (an-JEYE-nah PEK-toh-ris) is a sudden, severe chest pain that occurs when the heart does not receive enough oxygen and is usually brought on by emotional stress or physical exertion.

Murmurs may indicate some functional defect in the valves of the heart.

Coronary occlusion is a condition is which the heart does not receive enough blood due to blockage in a coronary artery.

Bradycardia (bray-dih-CAR-dee-ah) is an abnormally slow heartbeat (less than 60 beats per minute), and **tachycardia (tah-kih-CAR-dee-ah)** is an abnormally rapid heartbeat of 100 beats or more per minute.

Disorders of the Blood Vessels

Arteriosclerosis (ar-TEE-ree-oh-skler-OH-sis) is the thickening of the walls of the arteries. It is caused by a lack of elasticity and the calcification of connective tissue and fat deposits.

Gangrene results when an insufficient blood supply, due to disease or injury, causes the death of body tissue.

Phlebitis (fleh-BEYE-tis), is an inflammation of the lining of a vein accompanied by clotted blood. Symptoms include swelling, pain, and redness along the length of the vein.

Varicose veins were previously discussed in Chapter 4.

Hemorrhoids are varicosities in the walls of the lower rectum and the tissues around the anus.

Disorders of the Blood

Anemia is a deficiency in the number of red blood cells and/or the ratio percentile of hemoglobin in the blood resulting from a large or chronic loss of blood.

Iron-deficiency anemia is a condition caused by inadequate amounts of iron in the diet which may be corrected by iron supplements or foods that contain the mineral.

An **embolism** is a condition in which a foreign substance (embolus), such as air, a blood clot, cancer of fat cells, or bacterial clumps is carried by the bloodstream until it reaches an artery that is too small for passage.

Thrombosis is a blood clot that forms in a blood vessel or in the heart. It is caused by unusually slow blood circulation or blood and/or blood vessel changes, causing blood to remain stationary.

Hemophilia is a hereditary disease in which the blood clots too slowly to prevent excessive or prolonged bleeding.

Leukemia is a condition in which there is an overproduction of white blood cells which replace the red blood cells and interfere with the transport of oxygen to the tissues.

Sickle cell anemia is a chronic blood disease, inherited from both parents, that causes red blood cells to form in an abnormal shape. That results in the cells' inability to carry enough oxygen. Sickle cell anemia occurs most often in individuals of the black race. Cooley's anemia is the Mediterranean counterpart of sickle cell anemia.

Hematoma is a localized mass of blood found in an organ, tissue, or space as a result of injury that can cause a blood vessel to rupture.

AIDS

A discussion of AIDS should begin with an understanding of the terms associated with the subject. The terms most commonly used in conjunction with AIDS are as follows:

Acquired immune deficiency syndrome (AIDS)
Human immunodefiency virus (HIV)
AIDS related complex (ARC)
Sexually transmitted disease (STD)

It should be understood that AIDS is not the virus, but rather the immune system disorder that results from HIV infection.

As previously discussed, the immune system works to defend the body against infection. Especially important in this process are the following body parts and systems: the bone marrow, where lymphocytes (B and T cells) are manufactured; the thymus gland, where T cells mature; the lymphoreticular system, which provides storage sites for mature B and T cells; and the bloodstream, which contains cellular elements of the immune system.

Leukocytes, or white blood cells, are divided into two categories, lymphocytes and phagocytic cells. T-4 cells, a type of lymphocyte, trigger appropriate responses from other specialized white blood cells, such as activating the cells to produce antibodies.

> **NOTE:** Antibodies either neutralize an antigen or, along with other lymphocytes, adhere to the infected cells so that they can be destroyed.

A virus is the smallest disease-producing microorganism. It consists of genes surrounded by a protein layer and, by utilizing specific body cells, it is able to reproduce within the body. Some commonly known viral diseases are herpes, measles, polio, hepatitis, and AIDS.

One of the most difficult aspects of treating HIV infection is that the HIV virus is a retrovirus. This means that the virus uses the reproductive processes of the host cell (to which it becomes attached) to duplicate itself.

When HIV enters the bloodstream, it searches for a CD4 molecule to which it can attach itself. CD4 molecules are present on T-helper cells (among others), and very often the virus attaches itself to this specific cell. Once attached, these cells are considered target cells. The virus then sheds its outer covering of protein and enters the target cell through the area of attachment. The T cell signals the B cells to produce antibodies, while the HIV begins to convert RNA into viral DNA. Once converted, the altered DNA has the ability to pass into the nucleus of the target cell, where duplication begins. The newly formed viral particles are then released back into the bloodstream, where the process begins again, leaving destroyed T cells in its wake. This lowers the strength of the immune system, with the result that the body becomes susceptible to opportunistic diseases which can eventually cause death.

HIV is considered to be a weak virus when compared to polio; however, unlike polio, which has characteristics that respond to treatment, once HIV locks into the T cell in the bloodstream, it is nearly impossible to destroy.

According to the Florida Department of Health and Rehabilitation Services, HIV does not survive in an open environment (especially when subject to cold surfaces), drying, or ultraviolet light. It can be killed by soap, detergent, and alcohol; is not contracted from animals; and is not spread through casual contact. Kissing or contact with a person's tears, saliva, or sweat will not transmit the virus. The virus cannot live in food or drink. Coughing and sneezing will not transmit HIV because it is not an airborne virus. There is no risk from handling the linens of HIV- or AIDS-infected persons as long as there is no direct contact with their blood or bodily fluids.

The Stages of AIDS

Once HIV has entered the bloodstream and the immune response begins, antibodies will normally be produced within a range of two weeks to six months. The production of the antibodies is knows as seroconversion. At this point, HIV can be passed along to others.

The symptom stages from HIV to AIDS are as follows:

Stage 1—HIV infection: no physical indications of illness; antibodies to virus may be present.

Stage 2—ARC: chronic fatigue; unexplained chills, fever, or night sweats; 10 percent or greater weight loss without dieting; skin disorders; enlarged liver and/or spleen; swollen lymph glands; and chronic diarrhea.

Stage 3—AIDS: all of the above symptoms, as well as hair loss; skin and other cancers; pneumonia and other infections; and nerve and brain damage.

Individuals in the final stage of HIV infection (full-blown AIDS) usually exhibit the most severe characteristics of the disease.

Preventing AIDS

To date, there is no vaccine to prevent HIV infection, nor is there a cure for AIDS. Early intervention is the key to obtaining treatments that may be beneficial in improving the immune response and delaying the progression of the disease.

Those individuals who are at risk of contracting AIDS may be helped by eliminating all known cause of immune system suppression and by utilizing any and all therapies that stimulate immune system function. The correct diet, including vitamin, mineral, and herbal supplements; exercise; environment; and a proper mental attitude all attribute to the well-being of the immune system.

For more information about AIDS, call the AIDS Hotline: 1-800-342-2437.

In many states, professionals are currently required to attend an AIDS education course prior to licensure and license renewal, and in some cases, AIDS instruction has been added to school curriculum requirements.

Strict adherence to precautionary and sanitary measures in the workplace will assist in protecting the health and welfare of professionals and their clients.

Universal precautions should be followed at all times: however, most industries can benefit by customizing those precautions to suit their specific needs.

The following suggestions may serve as helpful reminders to professionals in the beauty care field:

- *Avoid accidents and practice all safety precautions applicable to the shop or salon.*
- *Wash hands with an antibacterial soap before and after each client.*
- *Always sanitize tools and implements before and after each client.*
- *Sanitize equipment, such has headrests, chair backs and arm rests, and facial, massage and manicure tables in between clients.*
- *Use disposable gloves whenever possible.*
- *If you cut, nick, or scrape yourself, treat the wound immediately and cover it.*
- *If you cut, nick, or scrape a client, apply gloves and treat the wound to the extent of your state board allowances and limitations.*
- *Avoid exposure and contact with another person's bodily fluids, especially blood.*
- *Attend available seminars and classes that provide updates on AIDS research.*
- *If you feel there is any chance that you may have contracted HIV, or if you simply wish to ease your mind, have an HIV antibody test performed. Keep in mind your responsibility to others and to yourself to minimize the risk of spreading this fatal disease.*

Review

Fill in the Blank

1. Blood is transported throughout the body through a _____ system.

2. Blood is a _____ tissue.

3. Blood is composed of _____, which is a _____ component, and _____, which are _____ components.

4. Blood cells include _____ cells, _____ cells, and _____.

5. Red blood cells carry _____ to the cells and _____ away from the cells.

6. _____ cells protect against disease by digesting bacteria that have invaded the body.

7. _____ assist in the clotting action of blood.

8. Plasma _____ and _____ blood cells.

9. The functions of the blood are _____, _____, _____, _____, and _____.

10. Blood is pumped through the blood vessels by the action of the _____.

11. The circulatory systems includes the _____ system.

12. There are two major blood circuits, _____ circulation and _____ circulation.

13. The general circulatory system carries blood _____ the rest of the body.

14. Pulmonary circulation carries blood _____ the heart to the _____ and back again.

15. The heart is a _____.

16. _____ should be performed only by individuals trained in CPR.

17. The heart can circulate about _____ gallons of blood per hour.

18. The right side of the heart carries _____ blood.

19. The left side of the heart carries _____ blood.

20. There are _____ chambers in the heart.

21. The upper chambers are known as _____ .

22. The lower chambers are called _____ .

23. _____ permit the blood to flow in only one direction and prohibit backflow.

24. The heartbeat generates the _____ .

25. Conduction cells send out _____ impulses.

26. _____ and _____ contractions are necessary to form a complete heartbeat.

27. The _____ is composed of one complete heartbeat.

28. The _____ is the largest artery in the body.

29. The _____ aorta carries blood to the arms, neck, and head.

30. The _____ aorta carries blood throughout the body.

31. The exchange of carbon dioxide and oxygen takes place in the _____ .

32. Veins carry deoxygenated blood _____ the capillaries to the heart via _____ .

33. _____ are a cell layer that connect arterioles with venules.

34. _____ molecules, _____ and _____ wastes can pass out of the capillaries.

35. Some conditions which may promote _____ are prolonged periods of standing or sitting; sitting with crossed legs; heredity; lack of exercise; being over-weight; pregnancy; and age.

36. _____ blood pressure is the pressure created at the moment of heart muscle con-traction.

37. Systolic blood pressure indicates the _____ level of blood pressure.

38. The force of blood in between beats is known as _____ pressure.

39. The blood pressure measuring device is called a _____ .

40. The sphygmomanometer measures the ratio of the _____ pressure to the _____ pressure.

41. A blood pressure reading of _____ is considered to be the most normal.

42. High blood pressure may lead to _____ or _____ .

43. Some services that may incur health risks to clients with high blood pressure are _____ , _____ , _____ , and _____ .

44. A _____ is an alternating expansion and contraction of an artery as blood flows through it.

45. The average pulse rate of an adult is _____ to _____ beats per minute.

46. Hemoglobin is a _____ found in red blood cells.

47. Fibrinogen is necessary for _____.

48. Electrolytes act as _____ buffers and maintain the _____ balance of the blood.

49. _____, _____, and _____ help the body control its chemical reactions.

50. Red blood cells are also known as _____.

51. White blood cells are known as _____.

52. Inflamation can occur through _____, _____, or the invasion of _____ bacteria.

53. Symptoms of inflammation include _____, _____, _____, and

    _____.

54. _____ is a combination of dead tissue, dead and living bacteria, dead leukocytes, and blood plasma.

55. Blood coagulation in humans should occur within _____ to _____ minutes.

56. Blood type is an _____ trait.

57. Blood type is determined by the presence or absence of the blood protein

    _____.

58. The four blood types are _____, _____, _____ and _____.

59–62. Identify the following blood types by whether agglutinogen is present individually, jointly, or not at all.

59.   A

60.   B

61.   AB

62.   O

63. The lymphatic system supplements the _____ system.

64. The _____ system consists of the lymph, lymph nodes and vessels, spleen, thymus gland, lymphoid tissue, and tonsils.

65. Lymph acts as an intermediary between blood in the _____ and the

    _____.

66. Lymph carries digested _____, _____, and _____ to the cells.

67. Lymph carries metabolic waste products _____ the cells.

68. Lymph vessels are located in most of the tissues and organs that have

    _____ .

69. The function of lymph nodes is to provide a site for _____ and to

    serve as a _____ .

70. _____ is an inherited, permanent immunity with which one is born.

71. _____ is the reaction that occurs as a result of exposure to disease-

    causing invaders of the body.

72. The two types of acquired immunity are _____ and _____ .

73. Immunization is the process of increasing an individual's resistance to a disease by

    _____ means.

74. When the body's immune system fails to protect itself against foreign materials and the

    antibodies that are formed irritate certain body cells, it is called _____ .

75. If a person is hypersensitive to a certain substance, he or she is considered to be

    _____ to the substance.

76. Symptoms of an _____ may include difficulty in breathing, dizziness,

    fainting, headache, swelling, rashes, inflammation, and nausea.

77. _____ disease is one of the leading causes of death.

78. _____ bacteria can cause acute rheumatic heart disease.

79. Any change from the normal rhythm of the heart action is known as _____ .

80. An irregular wrist pulse and abnormal heart rate are symptoms of

    _____ .

81. Symptoms of _____ include difficult or rapid breathing, swelling of organs,

    lung congestion, and coughing.

82. Sudden and severe chest pain brought on by emotional stress or physical exertion is a

    symptom of _____ .

83. Phlebitis symptoms include swelling, pain, and redness along the length of a _____ .

84. A deficiency in the number of red blood cells and/or the ration percentile of hemoglo-

    bin in the blood is known as _____ .

85. Inadequate amounts of _____ may produce a condition known as iron-deficiency

    anemia.

86. An _____ may exist in the form of air, a blood clot, cancer of fat cells, or bacte-

    rial clumps.

87. Hemophilia is a _____ disease.

88. An _____-production of white blood cells will interfere with the transport of oxy-

    gen to the tissues.

AIDS Review

89. AIDS stands for _____ .

90. AIDS is an immune system _____ .

91. The virus that causes AIDS is known as _____ , or

    _____ .

Matching

92–95. Match each term in column I with its description in column II.

Column I   *Column II*

_____ 92. Bone marrow   a. provides storage sites for mature B and T
                                           cells

_____ 93. Thymus gland   b. contains cellular elements of the immune
                                           system

_____ 94. Bloodstream   c. where B and T cells are manufactured

_____ 95. Lymphoreticular system   d. where T cells mature

Multiple Choice

96. Leukocytes are also known as: _____ .

    a. red blood cells   c. white blood cells
    b. target cells   d. infected cells

97. Antibodies may neutralize a/an: _____ .

    a. another antibody   c. arrhythmia
    b. anabolism   d. antigen

98. The smallest disease producing microorganism is a/an: _____ .

    a. molecule   c. spore
    b. virus   d. cell

99. The human immunodeficiency virus is a/an: _____ .

    a. retrovirus   c. restrictive virus
    b. introvirus   d. reticular virus

100. The number of symptom stages of HIV to AIDS is: _____ .

    a. two   c. four
    b. three   d. five

101. When HIV enters the bloodstream, it attaches itself to a: _____ .

    a. T cell   c. molecule
    b. T helpercell   d. CD4 molecule

102. B cells produce: _____ .
       a. toxins   c. virus
       b. antibodies   d. immunity

103. HIV converts RNA into viral: _____ .
       a. NNA   c. DNA
       b. ENA   d. TNA

Fill in the Blank

104. When the immune system is weakened, it becomes susceptible to _____ disease.

105. Once HIV has entered the bloodstream, antibodies may be produced in a range of _____ weeks to _____ months.

106. The production of antibodies is known as _____ .

107. Early intervention may be beneficial to improving the _____ response of the body.

108. Therapies should include those that _____ the immune system function.

The Respiratory System

The respiratory system is composed of organs that bring oxygen into the body and remove carbon dioxide through a three-stage process identified as external, internal, and cellular respiration, respectively. (Figure 6–1.)

External respiration (res-pih-RAY-shun), (meaning breathing or ventilation), is the exchange of oxygen and carbon dioxide between the body and the outside environment. The process consists of inhalation and exhalation. During inhalation, the air is warmed, moistened, and filtered on its passage to the air sacs (alveoli) of the lungs. Oxygen diffuses from this area of greater oxygen concentration to the bloodstream, and then into the red blood cells. The concentration of carbon dioxide becomes greater; it is diffused into the alveoli and then is expelled.

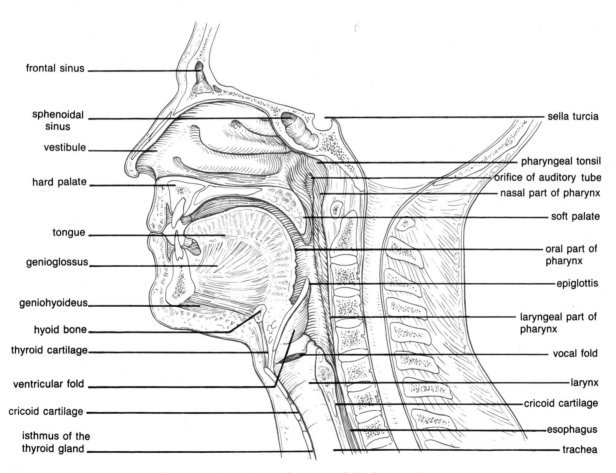

frontal sinus

sphenoidal sinus

vestibule

hard palate

tongue

genioglossus

geniohyoideus

hyoid bone

thyroid cartilage

ventricular fold

cricoid cartilage

isthmus of the thyroid gland

sella turcia

pharyngeal tonsil

orifice of auditory tube

nasal part of pharynx

soft palate

oral part of pharynx

epiglottis

laryngeal part of pharynx

vocal fold

larynx

cricoid cartilage

esophagus

trachea

Figure 6–1   Sagittal section of the face and neck

Internal respiration involves the exchange of carbon dioxide and oxygen between cells and the surrounding lymph and the oxidative process of energy in the cells. It is the difference between the concentrations of carbon dioxide and oxygen that governs the exchange which occurs between the air in the alveoli, the blood, and the tissue cells. Following inhalation, the alveoli transfer the new oxygen into the blood, which then results in the movement of oxygen into the tissue cells. During respiration, the tissue cells use up the oxygen, while simultaneously, they increase the carbon dioxide concentration, which then exceeds the level in the blood. The carbon dioxide then diffuses out of the cells and into the blood, which is now considered deoxygenated blood. The carbon dioxide is carried away to the lungs, where it is expelled during exhalation.

Cellular respiration (oxidation) is a chemical process within the cells by which oxygen is used to release energy that is stored in nutrient molecules, such as glucose. This energy may be released in the form of heat, to maintain body temperature, or may be used directly by cells for such work as the contraction of muscles. Following oxidation, the remaining waste products are transported from the cells through the circulatory system to the lungs, where they are exhaled.

Respiratory Organs and Structures

Air moves into the lungs through several passageways which include the nasal cavity, pharynx, larynx, trachea, bronchi, bronchioles, alveoli, lungs, pleura, and mediastinum. (See Figure 6–2.)

Nasal Cavity

When air enters the respiratory system through the nostrils, the air is filtered of dust and dirt particles, some bacteria, and some irritant fumes by cilia in the front of the nostrils. The air then moves into the nasal cavity, which is divided into right and left chambers by the septum, where the air is moistened by the mucus and warmed by blood vessels. Nerve endings (olfactory nerves) are located in the mucous membrane of the upper part of the nasal cavity which provide the sense of smell.

The sinuses are cavities of the skull in and around the nasal region lined with mucous membranes that aid in warming the air passing through them and provide resonance to the voice.

> **NOTE:** The unpleasant or "stuffed-up" voice sound indicative of a nasal cold is a result of blocked sinuses.

The Pharynx

After air leaves the nasal cavity, it enters the throat, or **pharynx (FAHR-inks)**, which serves as a common passageway for air and food, where it travels down on its way to the lungs. Adenoids and tonsils are lymphatic tissue which are located in this region, as well as the left and right eustachian tubes, which connect the middle ear.

The Larynx

The **larynx (LAHR-inks)**, or voice box, is a triangular chamber located below the pharynx that is composed of nine fibrocartilaginous plates. The largest of these plates

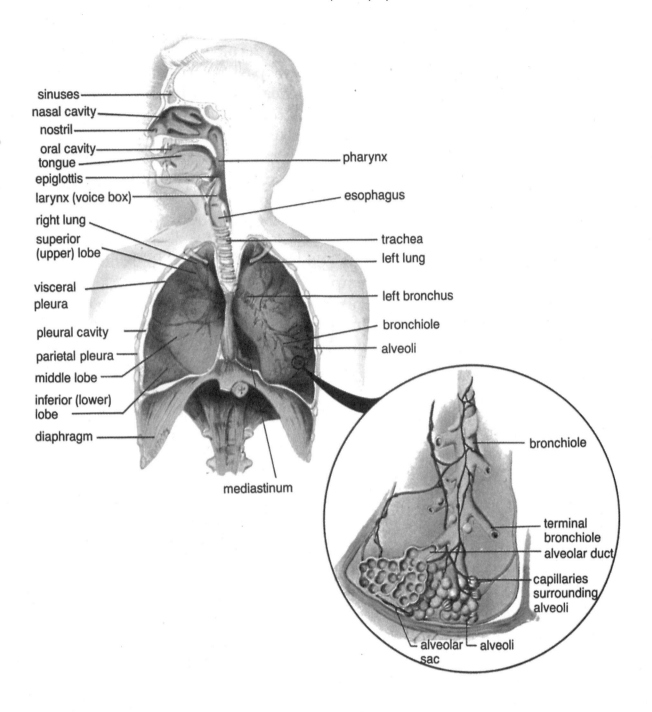

sinuses
nasal cavity
nostril
oral cavity
tongue
epiglottis
larynx (voice box)
right lung
superior
(upper) lobe
visceral
pleura
pleural cavity
parietal pleura
middle lobe
inferior (lower)
lobe
diaphragm

pharynx

esophagus

trachea
left lung

left bronchus

bronchiole

alveoli

mediastinum

bronchiole

terminal
bronchiole
alveolar duct

capillaries
surrounding
alveoli

alveolar
sac

alveoli

Figure 6–2   Respiratory organs and structures

is the **thyroid cartilage (THEYE-royd CAR-tih-lej)** or "Adam's apple." The larynx is lined with mucous membranes and houses the vocal cords. Tension on the vocal cords is exerted by muscles attached to the laryngeal cartilages. When lengthened, the vocal cords are relaxed and the voice is low-pitched; when shortened, they become tense and the voice is high-pitched.

The Trachea

The **trachea (TRAY-kee-ah)**, or windpipe, is a tube-like structure, approximately 4½ inches long, that extends from the larynx, passes in front of the esophagus, and continues on to form two bronchi, one for each lung. Alternate bands of membranes and 15 to 20 C-shaped rings of cartilage compose the tracheal wall. The C-shaped rings keep the trachea open for air passage to the lungs, although large pieces of food, tumors, or swollen lymph nodes in the neck may block the passage.

The function of the mucus in the trachea is to entrap inhaled dust particles. Cilia in the walls of the trachea then move dust-laden mucus upward to the pharynx, where it is eliminated through coughing or regurgitation.

The Bronchi, Bronchioles, and Alveoli

The lower end of the trachea divides into the right bronchus and the left bronchus, the right one being slightly shorter, wider, and more vertical in position than the left. As the bronchi enter the lungs, they subdivide, in Y-shaped forms, into the bronchial tubes and, then, the smaller, bronchioles. The bronchioles lead to an alveolar duct, which then ends in a cluster called alveolar sacs or alveoli.

It is in the moist walls within the alveoli and the capillaries that the exchange of carbon dioxide and oxygen takes place. In blood capillaries, carbon dioxide diffuses from red blood cells through the capillary wall into the alveoli, where it leaves to be exhaled through the nose and mouth. Oxygen is processed in the reverse as it is diffused from the alveoli into the capillaries and then into the red blood cells.

The Lungs

The lungs (pulmones) are two cone-shaped organs situated in the lateral chambers of the thoracic cavity, where they are separated by the mediastinum and the heart. The upper part of the lung is known as the apex; the lower part is considered the base and fits over the convex part of the diaphragm. Lung tissue is porous and spongy, due to the amount of air it contains. The right lung is larger and wider than the left (because the heart inclines to the left), but it is shorter due to the diaphragm's upward positioning on the right side to accommodate the liver. Due to its larger size, the right lung is divided into three lobes, superior, middle, and inferior, whereas the left lung is divided into two lobes, superior and inferior.

Each lung is enclosed in a double-walled sac of thin, moist membranes called pleura. Pleural fluid prevents friction while the two pleural membranes rub against each other during breathing. If the pleural cavity fills up with an excessive amount of serous fluid due to inflammation of the pleura (pleurisy), parts of the lung may collapse. Although breathing is not possible with a collapsed lung, the unaffected lung can continue the breathing process.

Mechanics of Breathing

Pulmonary ventilation of the lungs, or breathing, is the result of pressure changes in the chest cavity brought about by cellular respiration and mechanical breathing movements. Breathing allows the exchange of oxygen between the alveoli and the capillaries, followed by a subsequent exchange with the red blood cells. (See Figure 6–3.)

During inhalation, muscle fibers lift the ribs upward and outward, which increases thoracic cavity volume. Simultaneously, the diaphragm contracts, flattens, and moves downward, where pressure is exerted on the abdominal organs, increasing the vertical space within the chest cavity and decreasing the pressure. Atmospheric pressure is now greater, air rushes down to the alveoli and inhalation is complete.

Exhalation is a passive process in which the contracted muscles and the diaphragm relax and the opposite of the process of inhalation takes place: the ribs move down, the diaphragm moves up, the alveoli collapse, and the space in the cavity decreases, increasing the internal pressure and forcing air from the lungs.

Respiratory movements are the rhythmic movements of the rib cage while air is drawn in and expelled from the lungs. The combined processes of inhalation and

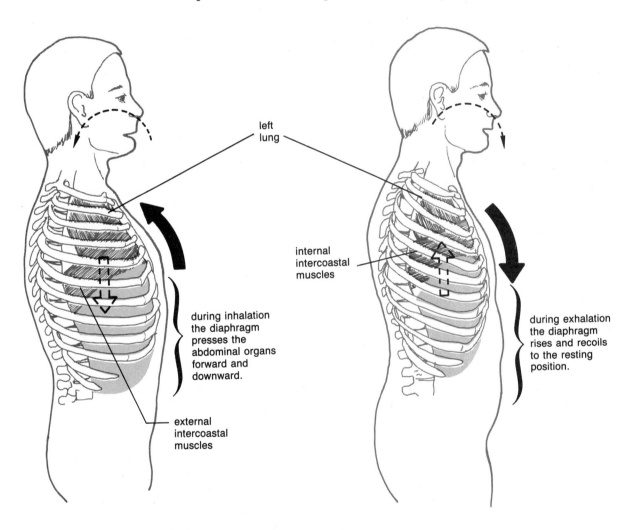

left
lung

internal
intercoastal
muscles

during inhalation
the diaphragm
presses the
abdominal organs
forward and
downward.

during exhalation
the diaphragm
rises and recoils
to the resting
position.

external
intercoastal
muscles

Figure 6–3   Mechanics of breathing—inhalation and exhalation

exhalation constitute one respiratory movement. The normal rate during quiet breathing in the average adult is 14 to 20 breaths per minutes (bpm). Respiratory rate can be affected by any of the following conditions: increased muscular activity or body temperature; pathological disorders (hyperthyroidism, specifically); gender (females, 16–20 bpm); age (birth, 40–60 bpm; 5 yrs., 24–26 bpm; 15 yrs., 20–22 bpm; 25 yrs. and over, 14–20 bpm); body position (prone, 12–14 bpm; sitting, 18 bpm; and standing, 20–22 bpm); and emotions.

The rate of breathing is controlled by independently functioning nervous and chemical factors. The respiratory center is divided into two subcenters, one for inhalation and the other for exhalation, and is located within the brain stem. It is primarily responsible for involuntary respiratory control, although it is not the only part of the brain that controls breathing. There is also a lung reflex (the Hering-Brewer reflex) that prevents overstretching of the lungs and sends nerve messages to the respiratory center for inhibition of inhalation and stimulation of exhalation.

The chemical control of respiration is dependent on the carbon dioxide levels in the blood. As blood circulates through the respiratory center, it becomes sensitive to increased carbon dioxide in the blood and the requirement for more oxygen. Hence, an individual performing vigorous exercise will breath more deeply and quickly.

Especially when working with chemicals, the professional should be aware of changes in the rate and the sounds of human respiration.

Eupnea (yoop-NEE-ah) *is normal breathing, with the usual quiet inhalations and exhalations.*

Apnea *is the temporary cessation of respiratory movements.*

Dyspnea (DISS-neeah) *is difficult, labored, or painful breathing in conjunction with discomfort and breathlessness.*

Hyperpnea (heye-per-NEE-ah) *is an increase in the depth and rate of breathing in conjunction with exaggerated respiratory movements.*

Orthopnea *is difficult or labored breathing when the body is in a prone position, which may be corrected by assuming a sitting or standing position.*

Polypnea *is rapid respiration or panting due to emotional trauma or increased muscular activity.*

Tachypnea (tak-eh-NEE-ah) *is an abnormally rapid rate of shallow breathing.*

Respiratory Disorders

It has been determined that the greatest loss in production hours each year is caused by the respiratory infection known as the common cold. Colds are usually the direct result of a virus and may often be the basis for more serious respiratory diseases because they lower the body's resistance to infection. Indirect causes of colds may include chilling, fatigue, and lack of a proper diet.

Infections and inflammations of the respiratory system can be caused by bacteria, viruses, or irritants.

Pharyngitis may be the result of bacteria, viruses, or irritants, including too much smoking or speaking, and is characterized by a red, inflamed throat, painful swallowing, and extreme dryness of the throat.

Laryngitis is an inflammation of the voice box that is often secondary to other respiratory infections. It results in hoarseness, loss of voice, sore throat, difficulty in swallowing, and throat dryness.

Tonsillitis is an infection of the tonsils, caused by bacteria, that tends to reoccur. Characteristics are severe sore throat, difficulty in swallowing, temperature, chills, and aching muscles.

Sinusitis is an infection of the mucous membranes accompanied by pain and nasal discharge.

Bronchitis is an inflammation of the mucous membrane of the trachea and the bronchial tubes. It may be acute or chronic in nature and is characterized by cough, fever, substernal pain, and rales (abnormal respiratory sounds).

It should be noted by the professional that acute bronchitis may be caused by the inhalation of irritating vapors. A shop or salon should always provide an adequate air filtration system for the safety and comfort of employees and clients alike. Special attention should be given to those areas of the establishment where chemical applications and nail tech services will be performed.

Pneumonia (noo-MOH-nyuh) is an infection of the lung(s), usually caused by bacteria, whereby the alveoli fill up with fluid. Onset is often sudden and is characterized by chills and chest pain.

Tuberculosis is an infectious disease usually occurring in the lungs. It may affect any organ or tissue of the body, however.

Diphtheria (dip-THEE-ree-ah) is a highly infectious disease that affects the upper respiratory tract and can be recognized by the formation of a grayish-white or yellow membrane on the pharynx, larynx, trachea, and/or tonsils. Diphtheria causes pain, swelling, and obstruction in this region; however, if the diptheria toxin is circulated through the bloodstream, it can lead to cardiac damage, fever, fatigue, paralysis, and death.

Whooping cough (pertussis) is an infectious disease characterized by repeated coughing attacks that end in a "whooping" sound. It can be fatal to infants. Respiratory ailments may also develop that are not associated with infectious causes.

Asthma (AZ-mah) is a respiratory disorder that may be triggered by emotional stress or the breathing of irritants. Symptoms include difficult breathing, wheezing, coughing, presence of mucus/sputum, and tightness in the chest. Emergency care may be required depending on the severity of the attack.

Emphysema (em-fih-ZEE-mah) is a noninfectious condition in which the lungs become overinflated, with the result that breathing is made difficult. No cure is currently known.

Cancer of the lungs is a malignant tumor which often forms in the bronchial epithelium and can be difficult to detect since the apparent symptoms are few. Many times, the condition is discovered during physical examinations that include chest x-rays. Surgery is often successful when the condition is diagnosed in its early stages.

Respiratory Distress Syndrome (RDS) is a condition most often affecting premature babies in which a false membrane forms within the alveoli, causing them to collapse.

6

Fill in the Blank

1. Organs bring _____ into the body and remove _____ from the body.

2. The three-stage process of respiration includes _____ , _____ , and _____ respiration.

3–9. Using _____ , _____ , or _____ , identify the following descriptions or characteristics with the type of respiration involved.

3. _____ The exchange of carbon dioxide and oxygen between cells and lymph.

4. _____ Involves the use of a chemical process in which oxygen is used to release energy.

5. _____ Exchange of oxygen and carbon dioxide between the body and the environment.

6. _____ The process consists of inhalation and exhalation.

7. _____ The aveoli transfer new oxygen into the blood.

8. _____ The air is warmed, moistened and filtered.

9. _____ Energy is released for use by the cells.

10. _____ moves into the _____ via the nasal cavity, pharynx, larynx, trachea, bronchi, bronchioles, alveoli, lungs, pleura and mediastinum.

11. The nostrils have the ability to _____ dust and dirt particles from the air.

12. Air is moistened by _____ and warmed by _____ .

13. Nerve endings are located in the _____ membrane.

14. _____ provide the sense of smell.

15. Sinuses aid in warming the air passing through them and provide _____ to the _____ .

16. The technical term for the voice box is _____ .

17. The largest plate in the larynx is known as the _____ cartilage or

    _____.

18. The larynx houses the _____.

19. When vocal cords are lengthened, they are _____ and the voice is

    _____-pitched.

20. When vocal cords are shortened, they are _____ and the voice is

    _____-pitched.

21. The trachea form _____ bronchi.

22. Membranes and C-shaped rings of cartilage compose the _____ wall.

23. _____ keep the trachea open for air passage to the lungs.

24. If breathing becomes obstructed due to choking, the _____ procedure

    should be used.

25. The exchange of carbon dioxide and oxygen takes place within the _____ and the

    _____.

26. Carbon dioxide diffuses from _____.

27. _____ is diffused from the alveoli.

28. The upper part of the lung is known as the _____.

29. _____ in lung tissue makes it porous and spongy.

30. The right lung is divided into _____ lobes; the left lung is divided into _____

    lobes.

31. Pleural fluid prevents _____ during the breathing process.

32. Breathing is the result of _____ in the chest cavity.

33. Pressure changes in the chest cavity are brought about by _____ and

    _____ breathing movements.

34. Atmospheric pressure is greater during _____.

35. _____ pressure forces air from the lungs.

36. The processes of inhalation and exhalation constitute _____ respiratory move-

    ment(s).

37. The normal rate of quiet breathing in the average adult is _____ to _____ breaths

    per minute.

38. _____ can be affected by increased muscular activity, body temperature,

    pathological disorders, and emotions.

39. _____ and _____ factors control the rate of breathing.

40. The respiratory center is located within the _____.

41. The respiratory center is primarily responsible for _____ respiratory control.

42. The lung _____ prevents the overstretching of the lungs.

43. Chemical control of respiration is dependent upon the level of _____ in the blood.

44. Professionals should be aware of the changes in the _____ and _____ of their client's breathing.

45. The common cold is usually the direct result of a _____.

46. Infections of the respiratory system may be caused by _____, _____, or _____.

47. Smoking may cause _____.

48. _____ is an inflammation of the voice box.

49. Tonsilitis is caused by _____.

50. Sinusitis is an infection of the _____.

51. _____ is an inflammation of the mucous membranes of the trachea and bronchial tubes.

52. Acute bronchitis may be caused by the inhalation of _____.

53. _____ is an infection of the lungs caused by bacteria.

54. Tuberculosis can affect any _____ or _____ of the body.

55. Diphtheria is a highly _____ disease.

56. Pertussis is also known as _____.

57. Asthma may be triggered from _____, _____, or the _____ of _____.

58. Emphysema causes _____ of the lungs.

59. _____ of the lungs is a malignant tumor, which often forms in the bronchial epithelium.

Matching

60–66. Match the following terms with their definitions.

60. _____	Apnea	a. normal breathing
61. _____	Dyspnea	b. increased depth and rate of breathing, with exaggerated movements
62. _____	Eupnea	c. Rapid respiration or panting due to emotional trauma/increased muscular activity
63. _____	Hyperpnea	d. temporary cessation of respiration

64. _____   Polypnea   e. abnormally rapid but shallow rate of breathing

65. _____   Tachypnea   f. difficult or labored breathing

66. _____   Orthopnea   g. difficult or labored breathing in a prone position

7

The Digestive System

Certain physical and chemical changes must occur before food can be rendered into a soluble, absorbable form that can be used by the cells.

Changing the complex insoluble food molecules into simple soluble molecules is necessary so that they can be transported by the blood to the cells and be absorbed through the cell membranes. This process is called digestion, or **enzymatic hydrolysis (EN-zeye-mah-tic heye-DRAW-lih-sis)**, and is accomplished by the action of a variety of digestive juices that contain **enzymes**. (Enzymes are chemical substances that promote chemical changes in living things without themselves being affected by the reactions.)

The digestive system consists of the **alimentary canal (al-ih-MENT-eh-ree)** (digestive or gastrointestinal tract) and **accessory digestive organs**. The organs are found in the head, thorax, abdomen, and pelvis, although most are concentrated in the abdomen. The digestive tract consists of the mouth, throat, esophagus, stomach, small intestine, large intestine (colon), and anus. These form a continuous tube—approximately 30 feet long when relaxed—from the mouth to the anus. However, during life, the tube measures only 12 to 15 feet due to its continual state of partial contraction.

Food within the digestive tract is not a part of the body and its cells until it is thoroughly digested so that the food molecules can pass through the small intestine into the bloodstream and then into the blood capillaries. It is at this point that the food molecules are diffused into the intestinal fluid and then into the body's tissue cells.

The teeth, tongue, salivary glands, pancreas, liver, and gallbladder are the accessory organs involved in the digestion process. (See Figure 7–1.)

When food enters the mouth, it is mechanically digested by the chewing and grinding action of the teeth. Chemical digestion of carbohydrates is initiated by the saliva, which contains an appropriate enzyme. The food then travels down the throat, through the esophagus, into the stomach (where protein digestion is initiated), and finally into the small intestine. The small intestine begins and finishes fat digestion and completes the digestion process of carbohydrates and proteins. The stomach and small intestine secrete digestive enzyme juices that chemically digest the food, changing the insoluble material into a soluble fluid substance, which is then transported into the bloodstream. As the soluble food molecules are circulated and absorbed through the blood capillaries and into the body cells, they are utilized for energy and the repair and the production of new cells. The undigested portion passes into the large intestine for elimination.

In addition to the intestinal juices, bile from the liver and pancreatic juice are required for digestion. Liver bile is needed for the digestion of fat, while the enzymes of pancreatic juices continue the digestion of protein, act on starch, and also digest

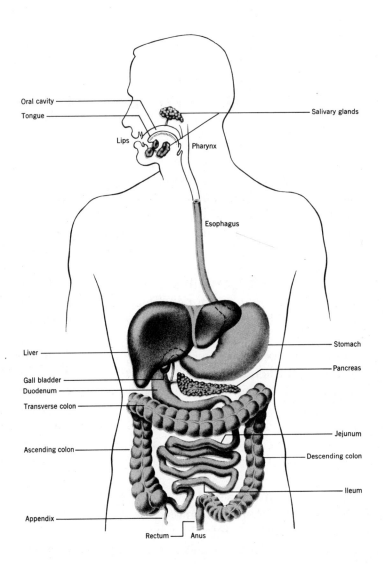

Figure 7-1   Alimentary canal and accessory organs

fat. The gallbladder is the storehouse of bile for the liver, releasing it as needed for the digestion of fats.

The functions of the large intestine are water absorption, nonpathogenic bacterial action, fecal formation, and defecation so as to regulate the body's water balance while storing and excreting the waste products of digestion.

Water is drawn from undigested food and indigestible materials that pass through the colon to be put back into the bloodstream, thus helping maintain the body's water balance.

Intestinal bacteria are nonpathogenic and act on the undigested food remains, turning them into acids, gases, and other waste products. Bacterial action also accounts for the formation of moderate amounts of B-complex vitamins and vitamin K, which is necessary for blood clotting.

Undigested or indigestible material in the colon contains water and remains in a liquid state until such time that it is converted into a semisolid mass through bacterial action and water absorption. Regular defecation can be promoted by regular exercise and by eating food containing bulk, such as whole grains, fruits, and vegetables.

The Role of Nutrients

In order for foods to be nutritious, they must contain the nutrients that are needed by the individual cells for proper cell functioning. These nutrients or substances are water, carbohydrates, lipids, proteins, vitamins, and minerals.

Water

Water is an essential component of all body tissues and serves several important functions in the body, which include acting as a solvent for all biochemical reactions, as a transport medium for substances, as a lubricant for joint movement and the digestive tract, as a control on body temperature (by evaporation from the pores of the skin), and as a cushion for organs, such as the brain and lungs.

Water constitutes between 55 and 65 percent of total body weight. Since water is continually lost through evaporation, excretion and respiration, it must continually be replaced. Some is replaced by drinking plain water; however, most of the body's water comes from ingested food.

Carbohydrates

Carbohydrates (car-boh-HEYE-drayts) are the main source of energy for the body. Excess carbohydrates, once converted into fat, can be stored in fat tissue until needed. There are some carbohydrates that should be minimized, such as sweets and soft drinks containing sugar, since they supply only calories. A better source is foods containing starches and cellulose, which provide energy, minerals, vitamins, and roughage.

Lipids

Lipids are a group of compounds that contain fatty acids with an alcohol. Fats are another source of energy and an essential nutrient to the maintenance of the body. They provide a source of energy during conditions of sickness or inadequate caloric intake, serve as a cushion for internal organs, insulate against cold, contribute to the formation of bile and steroid hormones, and contain fat-soluble vitamins. Total daily fat intake should not exceed 24 to 35 percent of the daily caloric intake.

Cholesterol is a common animal fat that is found in animal cell membranes. In the human skin, it is activated by sunlight to become vitamin D; in some people, however, it is also involved in the formation of arterial plaque, which blocks the passage of blood through the blood vessels and therefore can contribute to heart disease.

Proteins

As discussed in Chapter 1, proteins are essential to life. They provide the structure for all living things and are necessary components of hormones, enzymes, and genes. In order to exist and function, proteins require a certain balance and combination of **amino acids,** which are the chemical components of proteins. Amino acids serve the primary function of acting as transmitters for the central nervous system, which is essential for the brain to send messages or receive impulses. Amino acids are also responsible for the production of proteins and the ability of vitamins and minerals to perform their functions.

Protein substances are essential for the production and growth of organs, glands, nails, hair, muscles, ligaments, tendons, and certain body fluids.

Proteins have a more complex structure than carbohydrates or lipids and contain an amino group. Proteins serve a variety of functions in the body, such as enzymes that regulate the rate of chemical reactions and others that are important for the growth and repair of tissues. Proteins can also be used as a source of energy or aid various systems such as the hormonal, plasma transport, clotting, and antibody systems.

Protein in Foods Complete proteins are required for sustenance, as they provide the structure for all living things and participate in the chemical processes that promote life. Some vegetarian foods may be combined with others to create a complete protein combination, and thus may be used instead of animal protein for a well-balanced meal. For example, beans may be combined with any of the following to create a complete protein: cheese, corn, nuts, rice, sesame seeds, and wheat, whereas brown rice may be combined with beans, cheese, nuts, sesame seeds, or wheat.

> **NOTE:** Strict vegetarians must supplement their diets with B_{12} as this vitamin is almost exclusive to meat.

In the fruit group, apricots, avocados, bananas, cherries, figs, grapes, olives, papayas, and tomatoes contain 1 percent or more of protein. All soybean products, such as tofu and soy milk, are complete proteins. The only high-quality source of protein that is derived from animals is yogurt, which is made from milk that has been fermented using a mixture of yeast bacteria that are friendly to the digestive tract.

Vitamins

Vitamins contribute to good health by regulating the metabolism and assisting the biochemical processes that release energy from digested foods. Vitamins are considered micronutrients because they are required by the body in relatively small amounts as compared with requirements for carbohydrate, protein, fat, and water nutrients.

Vitamins are either water-soluble or oil-soluble in nature. Vitamins such as C and the B-complex vitamins are water-soluble and must be taken into the body daily, as they cannot be stored. Oil-soluble vitamins, such as A, D, E, and K, can be stored longer in the body's fatty tissue and in the liver.

Vitamins and minerals must be taken in their proper balance to insure the optimum functioning of all vitamins. Through synergy, combinations of two or more vitamins can create a stronger effect. For instance, bioflavanoids must be taken in conjunction with vitamin C in order to work properly. (See Tables 7–1, 7–2, and 7–3.)

Enzymes are chemicals that are essential to human bodily functions. They act as activators in the chemical reactions within the body and each fulfills a specific function. Vitamins work with enzymes, as **coenzymes**, to insure the expediency and accuracy of bodily activities. (See Table 7–4, page 139.)

Table 7-1   Supplements Needed for Assimilation of Vitamins

Vitamin Deficiency	Supplements Needed for Assimilation
Vitamin A	Choline, vitamins C, D, E, and F, zinc
Biotin	Folic acid, pantothenic acid (B5), B Complex, vitamins B12 and C
Choline	B complex, inositol, vitamin B12
Inositol	B complex, vitamin C
Niacin	B complex, vitamin C
PABA	B complex, folic acid, vitamin C
Pantothnenic acid	B complex, vitamins A, C, and E
Riboflavin (B2)	B complex, vitamin C
Thiamine (B1)	B complex, vitamins C and E, manganese
Vitamin B Complex	Calcium, vitamins C and E
Vitamin B6 (pyridoxine)	B complex, vitamin C, potassium
Vitamin C	Bioflavonoids, calcium, magnesium
Vitamin D	Calcium, choline, phosphorus, vitamins A, C, and F
Vitamin E	Inositol, manganese, selenium, vitamins A, B, C and F
Vitamin F	Vitamins A, C, D, and E
Vitamin K	Use natural sources (i.e., alfalfa, green leafy vegetables)

Table 7-2   Supplements Needed for Assimilation of Minerals

Mineral Deficiency	Supplements Needed for Assimilation
Calcium	Iron, magnesium, manganese, phosphorus, vitamins A, C, D, and F
Copper	Folic acid and cobalt, iron, zinc
Iodine	Iron, manganese, phosphorus
Magnesium	Calcium, phosphorus, potassium, vitamins B6, C, and D
Manganese	B complex, calcium, iron, vitamin E
Phosphorus	Calcium, iron, manganese, sodium, vitamin B6 (pyridoxine)
Silicon	Iron, phosphorus
Sodium	Calcium, potassium, sulfur, vitamin D
Sulfur	Biotin, pantothenic acid, potassium, vitamin B
Zinc	Calcium, copper, phosphorus, vitamin B6 (pyridoxine)

Table 7-3   Summary of Major Vitamins Needed in the Human Diet

VITAMIN	FOOD SOURCES	FUNCTION	DEFICIENCY DISEASES
A (Fat soluble)	Butter, fortified margarine, green and yellow vegetables, milk, eggs, liver	Night vision Healthy skin Proper growth and repair of body tissues	Night blindness Dry skin Slow growth Poor gums and teeth
B$_1$ (thiamine) (Water-soluble)	Chicken, fish, meat, eggs, enriched bread, whole grain cereals	Promotes normal appetite and digestion Needed by nervous system	Loss of appetite Nervous disorders Fatigue Severe deficiency causes beriberi
B$_2$ (riboflavin) (Water-soluble)	Cheese, eggs, fish, meat, liver, milk, cereals, enriched bread	Needed in cellular respiration	Eye problems Sores on skin and lips General fatigue
B$_3$ (niacin) (Water-soluble)	Eggs, fish, liver, meat, milk, potatoes, enriched bread	Needed for normal metabolism Growth Proper skin health	Indigestion Diarrhea Headaches Mental disturbances Skin disorders
B$_{12}$ (Cyanocobalamin) (Water-soluble)	Milk, liver, brain, beef, egg yolk, clams, oysters, sardines, salmon	Red blood cell synthesis Nucleic acid synthesis Nerve cell maintenance	Pernicious anemia Nerve cell malfunction
Folic Acid (Water-soluble)	Liver, yeast, green vegetables, peanuts, mushrooms, beef, veal, egg yolk	Nucleic acid synthesis Needed for normal metabolism and growth	Anemia Growth retardation
C (ascorbic acid) (Water-soluble)	Citrus fruits, cabbage, green vegetables, tomatoes, potatoes	Needed for maintenance of normal bones, gums, teeth, and blood vessels	Weak bones Sore and bleeding gums Poor teeth Bleeding in skin Painful joints Severe deficiency results in scurvy
D (Fat-soluble)	Beef, butter, eggs, milk	Needed for normal bone and teeth development Controls calcium and phosphorus metabolism	Poor bone and teeth structure Soft bones Rickets
E (tocopherol) (Fat-soluble)	Margarine, nuts, leafy vegetables, vegetable oils, whole wheat	Used in cell respiration Protects red blood cells from destruction	Anemia in premature infants No known deficiency in adults
K (Fat-soluble)	Synthesized by colon bacteria Green leafy vegetables, cereal	Essential for normal blood clotting	Slow blood clotting

ORGAN	JUICE	GLAND	ENZYME(S)	ACTION	ADDITIONAL FACTS
Mouth	Saliva	Salivary	Amylase found in ptyalin	Starch ⟶ Maltose	Physical as well as chemical hydrolysis Mucus flow starts here and continues throughout digestive tract
Esophagus	Mucus	Mucous	None	Lubrication of food	Peristalsis begins here
Stomach	Gastric juice along with HCL acid	Gastric	Protease, pepsin	Proteins ⟶ peptones and proteoses	Gastrin activates the gastric glands HCL supplies an acidic medium and kills bacteria Temporary food storage
Small intestine	Intestinal	Intestinal	Peptiadases	Peptones and proteoses amino acids	Absorption of end products occurs in small intestine
			Maltase	Maltose ⟶ glucose	Villi facilitates absorption
			Lactase	Lactose ⟶ glucose and galactose	
			Sucrase	Sucrose ⟶ glucose and fructose	
			Lipase	Fats ⟶ fatty acids and glycerol	
	Bile	Liver	None	Emulsifies fat	Neutralizes stomach acid
	Pancreatic	Pancreas	Protease (trypsin)	Proteins ⟶ peptones, and amino acids	Secretin stimulates the flow of pancreatic juice
			Amylase (amylopsin)	Starch ⟶ maltose	
			Lipase (steapsin)	Fats ⟶ fatty acids and glycerol	
			Nucleases	Nucleic acids (DNA/RNA) nucleotides	

Minerals

Minerals are natural chemical elements found in the earth that, like vitamins, function as coenzymes. Minerals are necessary for the proper composition of body fluids, the formation of blood and bone, and the maintenance of healthy nerve function.

Minerals are obtained from the inorganic compounds in food and are necessary for normal growth and maintenance. (See Table 7–5.)

Table 7-5   Summary of Essential Minerals and Trace Elements Needed for Health

MINERAL	FOOD SOURCES	FUNCTION	DEFICIENCY DISEASES
Calcium	Milk, cheese, dark green vegetables, dried legumes, sardines, shellfish	Bone and tooth formation Blood clotting Nerve transmission	Stunted growth Rickets Osteoporosis Convulsions
Chlorine	Common table salt, seafood, milk, meat, eggs	Formation of gastric juices Acid-base balance	Muscle cramps Mental apathy Poor appetite
Chromium	Fats, vegetable oils, meats, clams, whole-grain cereals	Involved in energy and glucose metabolism	Impaired ability to metabolize glucose
Copper	Drinking water, liver, shellfish, whole grains, cherries, legumes, kidney, poultry, oysters, nuts, chocolate	Constituent of enzymes Involved with iron transport	Anemia
Fluorine	Drinking water, tea, coffee, seafood, rice, spinach, onions, lettuce	Maintenance of bone and tooth structure	Higher frequency of tooth decay
Iodine	Marine fish and shellfish, dairy products, many vegetables, iodized salt	Constituent of thyroid hormones	Goiter (enlarged thyroid)
Iron	Liver, lean meats, legumes, whole grains, dark green vegetables, eggs, dark molasses, shrimp, oysters	Constituent of hemoglobin Involved in energy metabolism	Iron-deficiency anemia
Magnesium	Whole grains, green leafy vegetables, nuts, meats, milk, legumes	Involved in energy conversions and enzyme function	Growth failure Behavioral disturbances Weakness Spasms
Phosphorus	Milk, cheese, meat, fish, poultry, whole grains, legumes, nuts	Bone and tooth formation Acid-base balance Involved in energy metabolism	Weakness Demineralization of bone
Potassium	Meats, milk, fruits, legumes, vegetables	Acid-base balance Body water balance Nerve transmission	Muscular weakness Paralysis
Selenium	Fish, poultry, meats, grains, milk, vegetables (depending on amount in soil)	Necessary for vitamin E function	Anemia Increased mortality?
Sodium	Common table salt, seafood, most other foods except fruit	Acid-base balance Body water balance Nerve transmission	Muscle cramps Mental apathy
Sulfur	Meat, fish, poultry, eggs, milk, cheese, legumes, nuts	Constituent of certain tissue proteins	Related to deficiencies of sulfur-containing amino acids
Zinc	Milk, liver, shellfish, herring, wheat bran	Involved in many enzyme systems Necessary for vitamin A metabolism	Growth failure Lack of sexual maturity Impaired wound healing Poor appetite

NOTE: Certain vitamins, minerals, and enzymes belong to a group known as **antioxidants**. Antioxidants assist in protecting the body from **free radicals** (cell-damaging atoms). By damaging the cells, free radicals inhibit the immune system which, in turn, creates a vulnerability to infections and disease. Certain enzymes that occur naturally in the body neutralize the free radicals, but at times, supplements such as vitamins A, E, and C are required for optimum health.

Dietary Guidelines

The Recommended Daily Allowance (or RDA) was established over 40 years ago to indicate the daily amount of vitamins necessary to prevent disease. This allowance, however, provides only the minimum necessary to ward off such diseases as rickets, scurvy, beri beri, and night blindness, rather than addressing what is required to maintain optimum health. An Optimum Daily Allowance plan provides a better vehicle for maintaining health and can be customized to suit the individual's needs. Nutritional counseling is the most conscientious approach to formulating individual diets and supplement needs.

The following guidelines were established to help prevent the most prevalent and devastating diseases in our society, namely, diabetes, cancer, hypertension, and heart disease:

1. Eat a variety of foods.
2. Maintain a desirable weight.
3. Avoid too much fat (especially saturated fat) and cholesterol.
4. Eat foods with adequate starch and fiber.
5. Avoid too much sugar and sodium.
6. Avoid too many alcoholic beverages.

Conditions such as pregnancy, disease, emotional stress, and old age must be considered when determining daily individual dietary requirements. Nutritional requirements may vary for a variety of reasons, including the methods used to process, store or cook foods; malabsorption disorders; and the individual's internal environment.

Foods and Food Processing

Overcooked foods have been proven to be potentially carcinogenic when ingested. This is due to the agents and chemical changes that occur when bread crust is toasted or meat is charcoal grilled. Nitrogenous substances are consumed when individuals eat fried pork or bacon. Fat, protein, and other organic compounds contained in animals that are used as a meat source undergo changes in chemical structure when cooked at extreme temperatures. These toxic chemical changes put the individual at risk for cancer.

Certain foods, such as soybean products and peanuts, should be consumed in moderation since they contain certain enzyme inhibitors. Too many legumes can create excessive gas and discomfort and may be difficult to digest. Nuts should be fresh rather than roasted, and exposure to air and light should be avoided.

Fruits and vegetables lose nutrients while being stored or when overripe, and therefore contain more vitamins and enzymes when fresh. Additionally, organically grown foods are the healthiest since they are grown without the use of pesticides, insecticides, or growth-inducing chemicals.

Vitamins and enzymes are extremely sensitive to heat and will be destroyed in the cooking process. Canned, processed, and boxed foods should not be used and steam cooking should be minimized to protect vitamin and enzyme content. Frozen foods are the next best substitute to fresh foods; fruit and vegetables should be eaten raw whenever possible.

Table salt can be detrimental to the body's systems in many ways and may cause changes in the fluid and mineral balance of the body. An excessive amount of salt in the system may create fluid build-up and hydrostatic pressure in the tissues, often leading to high blood pressure, heart disease, or stroke. Salt does not allow the blood to circulate properly and inhibits the process of waste excretion, a process that is especially important in cases of disease for the release of toxins, metabolic wastes, gases, and bacteria.

The ingestion of sugar may lead to many disorders and is an influential factor in many diseases. Refined carbohydrates (sugar) stimulate the pancreas to produce insulin, a substance necessary to the metabolization of simple carbohydrates. The more simple the carbohydrates ingested, the more insulin the pancreas must produce. This can result in the overstimulation of the pancreas which can damage this important gland, resulting in diabetes. Excess ingestion of refined simple carbohydrates can also lead to hypoglycemia, a condition in which the body is unable to metabolize the sugar properly. This inability to metabolize leads to fatigue, dizziness, confusion, headache, and other symptoms and may eventually result in the collapse of the adrenal glands, which are necessary in order to handle stress.

Simple carbohydrates should be eliminated from the diet; however, complex carbohydrates, such as fruits, vegetables, beans and natural whole grains, should be included. Complex carbohydrates provide a steady source of energy for the body.

Aluminum cooking utensils should never be used in the cooking process because foods cooked in aluminum produce a chloride poison that neutralizes digestive juices and produces acidosis and ulcers. Aluminum enters the body in many forms, from antacids (aluminum hydroxide content) and pain/inflammation drugs (over-the-counter) to feminine douche preparations. Research has shown that an accumulation of aluminum salts in the brain is a factor in seizures and reduced mental faculties. Current studies link Alzheimer's disease with excessive accumulations of aluminum in the nerve cells of the brain, which prevents the nerves impulses from functioning properly. Aluminum is also excreted by the kidneys and toxic amounts may impair kidney function.

In addition to the previously mentioned products, aluminum is found in the following substances and items and should be avoided when possible: shampoos (aluminum lauryl sulfate), foil, most city water, food-processing ingredients (especially in pickles and relishes), baking powder, antiperspirants/deodorants, beer (especially in cans), bleached flour, table salt, tobacco smoke, cream of tartar, Parmesan and grated cheeses, and canned goods. Lovers of "fast foods" should know that processed cheese has a high aluminum content which gives the cheese its melting quality for use on hamburgers.

Eating Disorders

Obesity (oh-BEE-sih-tee) is one of the most common nutritional diseases in our society. By definition, an obese person is one who has excess body fat and weighs 15 to 20 percent more than the maximum body weight for his or her particular gender, height, age, and bone structure. Obesity can affect physical and mental health, often seriously. Heart disease, high blood pressure, forms of diabetes, kidney problems, complications during pregnancy, and liver damage can occur either separately or in conjunction with each other, causing additional stress on the body and its systems. The psychological effects of obesity can lead to depression, insecurity, low self-esteem, and a variety of other disorders. Recently, obesity has been linked to food sensitivity or allergies in some cases. Additionally, an inadequate intake of the essential nutrients needed for the performance of body organs may increase the tendency to obesity. Other causes of obesity include glandular malfunctions, malnutrition, emotional tension, boredom, and poor eating habits.

Anorexia nervosa (an-er-EK-see-ah ner-VOH-sa) appears to be more psychologically oriented than many cases of obesity, which can be linked to overeating or eating habits. In true anorexia nervosa there is no real loss of appetite, but rather a refusal to eat due to an unrealistic idea of one's body image and a fear of weight gain. The American Psychiatric Association has identified the following criteria for the diagnosis of anorexia nervosa:

1. Fear of becoming obese that does not diminish with weight loss.
2. Distorted body image, such as claiming to be or feeling overweight even when emaciated.
3. Weight loss of at least 25 percent of original body weight.
4. Refusal to maintain minimal body weight.
5. No known illness that accounts for weight loss.
6. Cessation of menstruation.

Bulimia (byu-LEE-mee-ah) is another eating disorder that is associated with a fear of weight gain and is characterized by episodic binge eating, followed by purging behavior.

The treatment of anorexia nervosa and bulimia is difficult and lengthy, involving the resolution of the underlying psychological problems and disorders. Early detection and intervention are essential due to the irreversible damage that will occur to tissues and homeostatic balances if the disorder is left untreated.

Disorders of the Digestive System

There are many common disorders that interfere with the digestive system of the human body but can be controlled with diet and proper nutrition.

Hiatal (heye-AY-tal) hernia is a rupture that occurs when the stomach protrudes above the diaphragm through the esophagus opening. This may cause the condition known as heartburn, which can usually be relieved with a change of diet. Surgery is seldom required.

Heartburn is a condition that results from the backflow of the highly acidic gastric juices into the lower end of the esophagus which irritates the lining, causing a burning sensation. Ingesting a solution of bicarbonate of soda will neutralize the stomach's gastric juices and give temporary relief.

Gastritis (gah-STREYE-tis) is an acute or chronic inflammation of the stomach's mucous membrane lining caused by spicy food or some drugs. Gastritis is subdivided into three categories. **Atrophic (ay-TROH-fik) gastritis** is a chronic form in which the membrane has atrophied, **corrosive gastritis** is an acute form caused by corrosive poisons, and **infectious gastritis** is an acute form associated with infectious diseases.

Peptic ulcers are lesions that occur in either the stomach or the small intestine as the result of insufficient mucus secretion and an oversecretion of gastric juice. Psychological stress can contribute to the development of peptic ulcers. The pain accompanying peptic ulcers may be relieved by ingesting bicarbonate of soda.

Enteritis (en-ter-EYE-tis) is an inflammation of the intestine caused by a bacterial, viral, or protozoan infection, food poisoning, or an allergic reaction to certain foods.

Colitis is a condition in which the colon becomes inflamed and is accompanied by excessive mucus secretion.

Appendicitis is the inflammation of the veriform appendix.

Infectious hepatitis is a viral infection of the liver caused by contaminated food or water. Symptoms include chills, fever, jaundice, fatigue, and gastrointestinal disturbances.

Serum hepatitis is an inflammation of the liver caused by a virus found only in the blood. It may be transmitted by a blood transfusion contaminated with the virus or through the use of inadequately sterilized needles or surgical equipment. Evidence indicates that transmission via semen and respiratory secretions can occur.

Cirrhosis (seh-ROH-sis) is a chronic and progressive inflammation of the liver commonly caused by excessive alcohol consumption.

Gallstones are deposits of crystallized cholesterol that form in the gallbladder. They can block the bile duct, causing pain and digestive disorders. Large gallstones must be surgically removed.

The digestive system and its functions fully impact the general and specific health of an individual. From the smallest elements, such as amino acids, to the actual organs and structures, the digestive system works in unison to revitalize the body and its cells on a continual basis. It is a potentially sensitive system that requires all its components to function at optimum performance. A deficiency in vitamins or enzymes will cause disharmony and the malfunctioning of other components. Nerve impulses are helped or hindered by substances that are ingested into the system. Muscles and tendons require protein to reproduce the cells needed for performance. The skin, hair, and nails all reflect an individual's internal health, as do the glands and organs.

Professionals are exposed daily to these health indicators and, therefore, should be aware of the contributing factors involved. Client consultations are essential in providing the professional with the information needed in order to determine whether a service should be performed. Additionally, during conversations with clients, it is perfectly acceptable to share what you know about the importance of nutrition and how it affects the body as long as you do not diagnose or prescribe.

The importance of good nutrition and the proper use of supplements cannot be overstressed. As trained professionals, the importance may be obvious, but the application is another one of those "easier said than done" situations. For instance, think back over the past two weeks and note the number of times you started the day off with a good breakfast—or had the option of taking time for lunch. Maybe you did have (or take) time for one meal or the other, but what was the condition in which you had to satisfy the reasonable fuel demands of your body: a bagel in the car on the way to work—two bites of a burger in between clients—or a chemical-laden microwave quick-fix? This is rather embarrassing—not to mention down-right unhealthy—for individuals who have been trained to know better!

Remember those first theory classes in cosmetology, barbering, esthetician, or massage school? Far too often, the demands of our profession require that we put our own health in jeopardy, all for the want of time to ingest good, nourishing food.

It is an obvious requirement and responsibility of our industry to serve the clients and, in many cases, to put them first. However, we also have a responsibility to ourselves to maintain good health, and in order to do so, we must give some priority to our bodies' nutritional requirements.

Realize that everything that is ingested affects the body in some way, whether good or bad, minimally or optimally. Some quick research or an appointment with a nutritional specialist can point you in the right direction to determining your nutritional needs. A recommended text is James F. Balch, M.D., and Phyllis A. Balch, C.N.C., Prescription for Nutritional Healing.

Fill in the Blank

1. Before food can be used by the cells, certain _____ and _____ changes must take place.

2. Complex insoluble food molecules must be changed into _____ molecules.

3. _____ is the technical term for digestion.

4. Digestive juices contain _____.

5. Enzymes are chemical substances that promote _____ in living things.

6. Enzymes are _____ affected by the chemical reactions they create.

7. The digestive system consists of the _____ canal and _____ digestive organs.

8. The alimentary canal is also known as the _____ or _____ tract.

9–18. Identify the following body structures as being part of the alimentary canal or as being an accessory digestive organ.

9. _____ mouth   14. _____ large intestine

10. _____ tongue   15. _____ stomach

11. _____ liver   16. _____ abdomen

12. _____ small intestine   17. _____ throat

13. _____ pancreas   18. _____ esophagus

19. Food cannot be considered part of the body and its cells until it is _____.

20. Food is _____ digested by the action of the teeth.

21. _____ initiates the chemical digestion of carbohydrates.

22. Fat digestion begins and ends in the _____ intestine.

23. After food has been changed into a soluble fluid substance, it is transported into the _____.

24. Soluble food molecules are utilized for _____ , _____ , and the _____ of new cells.

25. Indigestible substances pass into the _____ intestine.

26. In addition to intestinal juices, _____ and _____ are needed for digestion.

27. Liver bile is required for the digestion of _____ .

28. Pancreatic juice enzymes assist in the digestion of _____ , _____ , and _____ .

29. The gallbladder stores _____ for the liver.

30. _____ absorption is one function of the large intestine.

31. Intestinal bacteria are _____ .

32. Bacterial action turns undigested food remains into _____ , _____ , and other _____ .

33. The formation of _____ vitamins and vitamin _____ are a result of bacterial action.

34. _____ is necessary for blood clotting.

35. The nutrients, or substances, necessary for proper cell functioning are _____ , _____ , _____ , _____ , _____ , and _____ .

36. All body tissues require the essential element of _____ .

37. Water constitutes between _____ and _____ percent of total body weight.

38. Most of the body's water comes from ingested _____ .

39. The main source of energy for the body comes from _____ .

40. Foods containing starches and cellulose provide _____ , _____ , _____ , and _____ .

41. _____ contain fatty acids with an alcohol.

42. Another source of energy that also serves as a cushion for the body are _____ .

43. Cholesterol is an animal fat that, when in the human skin, is activated by sunlight to become _____ .

44. Cholesterol may cause the formation of _____ .

45. Proteins are necessary components of _____ , _____ , and _____ .

46. Proteins are comprised of _____ .

47. Proteins require a balance and _____ of amino acids.

48. Amino acids act as _____ for the central nervous system.

49. Amino acids aid _____ and _____ to perform their functions.

50. Proteins have a more _____ structure than carbohydrates or lipids.

51. Strict vegetarians should supplement their diet with _____.

52. Vitamins regulate _____ and assist in _____ processes.

53. Vitamins are considered to be _____.

54. Vitamins may be _____-soluble or _____-soluble.

55. Vitamins _____ and _____ cannot be stored in the body.

56. The combination of two or more vitamins to create stronger vitamin function is known as _____.

57. _____ act as activators in chemical reactions.

58. Each enzyme has a _____ in the body.

59. Minerals and vitamins function as _____.

60. Minerals are necessary for the proper composition of _____.

61. The formation of blood and bone requires _____.

62. Minerals assist in the maintenance of healthy _____ function.

63. Minerals are obtained from _____ compounds in food.

64. Vitamins, minerals, and enzymes that protect the body from free radicals are known as _____.

65. Free radicals are _____ that cause damage to cells.

66. The RDA provides the _____ daily amount of vitamins.

67. Fats and proteins undergo _____ changes when cooked at extreme temperatures.

68. Foods that are grown without the use of pesticides, insecticides, or growth-inducing chemicals are known as _____ foods.

69. Vitamins and enzymes are sensitive to _____.

70. _____ foods are the next best substitute for fresh foods.

71. Excessive salt in the system may lead to _____, _____, and _____.

72. Salt does not allow the blood to _____ properly and inhibits the process of waste excretion.

73. The overstimulation of the pancreas to produce insulin wears out the _____.

74. _____ is a condition in which the body cannot metabolize sugar properly.

75. _____ carbohydrates provide a source of energy for the body.

76. Using aluminum cooking utensils produces a _____ poison.

77. Aluminum may enter the body through the use of _____ and _____ drugs.

78. An accumulation of aluminum in the _____ of the brain prevents the nerve cells from functioning properly.

79. _____ is a common nutritional disease.

80. Some conditions of obesity have been linked with food _____ or _____ .

81. Anorexia nervosa is more _____ oriented than many cases of obesity.

82. _____ is associated with a fear of weight gain.

83. Many disorders of the digestive system can be controlled with _____ and proper _____ .

Matching

84–95. Match the following disorders with their descriptions.

84. _____ Hiatal hernia   a. lesions that appear in the stomach or small intestine

85. _____ Gastritis   b. results from the backflow of acidic juices

86. _____ Heartburn   c. rupture associated with stomach protrusion

87. _____ Atrophic gastritis   d. inflammation of the stomach's mucous membrane

88. _____ Peptic ulcers   e. chronic atrophy of the membrane

89. _____ Enteritis   f. deposits of crystallized cholesterol

90. _____ Colitis   g. caused by excessive alcohol consumption

91. _____ Appendicitis   h. caused by food poisoning or an allergic food reaction

92. _____ Infectious hepatitis   i. an inflamed colon

93. _____ Serum hepatitis   j. inflammation of the appendix

94. _____ Cirrhosis   k. viral infection of the liver caused by food or water

95. _____ Gallstones   l. inflammation of the liver caused by a virus found in blood

The Elimination of Waste

8

Food is utilized through the processes of digestion, absorption, and metabolism which separate digestible substances from undigestible ones. Waste products formed by the total process are then excreted; if the metabolic wastes and undigested food were left to accumulate in the body, they would act as toxins, or poisons.

The Excretory System

Elimination takes place through a process that includes the kidneys, skin, intestines, and lungs. The lungs provide the excretory function of giving off carbon dioxide and water vapor. The urinary system is an excretory agent of nitrogenous wastes, salts, and water, and the skin functions in the excretion of dissolved wastes (mostly dissolved salts) through the process of perspiration. The intestines excrete indigestible residue, water, and bacteria. (See Table 8–1.)

The Urinary Tract

The urinary system, consisting of two kidneys, two ureters, a bladder, and a urethra, performs the main excretory function of the body. The most important excretory organs are the kidneys, which function in the removal of nitrogenous waste products. If the kidneys do not function properly, toxic wastes will accumulate in the cells, which will literally poison themselves.

The kidneys are bean-shaped organs located against the dorsal wall of the abdominal cavity and on either side of the vertebral column. The right kidney is displaced to a position slightly lower than the left kidney by the liver. The kidneys are complex structures consisting of blood vessels, fat tissue, fibrous tissue, arteries, veins, and tubular branches and loops. Kidney nephrons form urine through three processes: filtration, reabsorption, and secretion.

Filtration is the first step, whereby blood from the renal artery travels from its

Table 8–1   Elimination of Waste Products

ORGAN	PRODUCT OF EXCRETION	PROCESS OF ELIMINATION
Lungs	carbon dioxide and water vapor	exhalation
Kidneys	nitrogenous wastes and salts dissolved in water to form urine	urination
Skin	dissolved salts	perspiration
Intestines	solid wastes and water	defecation

151

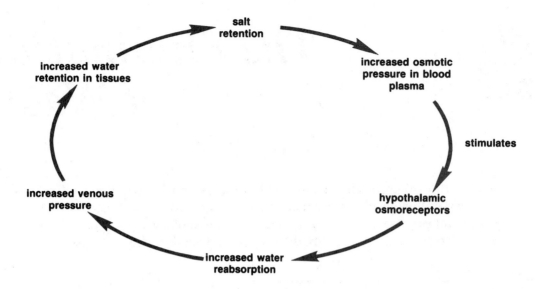

Figure 8–1   How salt retention influences water retention in tissues

origin to small capillaries of the glomerulus. During the course of travel, blood vessels become increasingly narrow, which results in an increase in blood pressure. This high blood pressure forces fluid (nephric filtrate), consisting of water, glucose, amino acids, salts, and urea, to filter from the blood.

Reabsorption is the process that follows the filtration process of the absorbing of useful substances and water by the capillaries. In addition to water, the substances include glucose, amino acids, vitamins, bicarbonate ions, and the chloride salts of calcium, magnesium, sodium, and potassium.

The proximal tubules reabsorb about 80 percent of the water filtered out of the blood in a process known as obligatory water absorption, which occurs by osmosis. Simultaneously, the other useful substances are being transported back into the blood. In the distal convoluted tubules, 10 to 15 percent of the water is reabsorbed back into the bloodstream by the process of optional absorption. This function is controlled by **antidiuretic hormone (an-tee-deye-eh-REH-tik)** (ADH), which helps maintain the balance of bodily fluids by controlling the reabsorption of water. (See Figure 8–1.)

Secretion (seh-KREE-shun) is the opposite of reabsorption and involves the transport of substances from the blood in the capillaries into the urine. Substances secreted into the urine include ammonia, hydrogen ions, potassium ions, and some drugs.

Urine passes from the kidneys and eventually travels down the ureter into the urinary bladder, a hollow muscular organ made of elastic fibers that acts as a reservoir, until about one pint has been accumulated. Emptying the bladder takes place by involuntary muscular contractions that can be somewhat controlled through the nervous system. Urinary secretion is also influenced by chemical control during the reabsorption process due to the hormones involved in that stage.

Disorders of the Excretory System

Acute kidney failure may be the result of shock, injury, bleeding, poisoning, or sudden heart failure. A common symptom is the absence of urine formation (anuria) which, if it continues, will lead to **uremia (yoo-REE-mee-ah),** a toxic condition in which the blood retains urinary waste products because the kidneys fail to excrete them. Symptoms include headaches, nausea, vomiting, and, in extreme cases, coma and death. Hemodialysis is the process by which an artificial kidney machine is used to remove waste products from the kidneys.

Cystitis (sis-TEYE-tis) is an inflammation of the mucous membrane lining of the urinary bladder (caused by bacterial infection or kidney inflammation) that has spread to the bladder. Proper treatment involves antibiotics to kill the bacteria causing the inflammation.

Dysuria (dish-YOO-ree-ah) is difficult or painful urination. **Incontinence** occurs when an individual loses voluntary control over urination, resulting in voiding whenever the bladder fills.

Kidney stones are microscopic crystals of calcium phosphate that clump together when stagnation of urine occurs, eventually blocking the urine flow in the ureter. Extended immobility, dehydration, renal infection, and an overactivity of hormonal secretion that regulates blood calcium levels may cause the formation of kidney stones. Treatment may involve causing the stones to pass, dissolving the stones, or surgical removal.

Review

Fill in the Blank

1. The processes of digestion, absorption, and metabolism separate _____ substances from _____ substances.

2. If metabolic wastes were allowed to remain in the body, they would act as _____.

3. The process of elimination includes the involvement of the _____, _____, _____, and _____.

4. The lungs excrete _____ and _____.

5. The _____ excretes nitrogenous wastes, salts, and water.

6. The skin excretes dissolved wastes through _____.

7. The _____ excrete indigestible residue, water, and bacteria.

8. The kidneys are the most important _____ organs.

9. _____ is formed through the processes of filtration, reabsorption, and secretion.

10. High _____ forces are used during filtration to extract substances from the blood.

11. Reabsorption is the process of absorbing _____ substances and _____ after the filtration process.

12. Obligatory water absorption occurs by _____.

13. An _____ hormone controls the reabsorption of water.

14. Secretion is the _____ of reabsorption.

15. Secretion transports substances from the _____ into the urine.

16. The urinary bladder acts as a _____.

17. Urinary secretion can be somewhat controlled through the _____ system.

18. Shock, injury, bleeding, poisoning, or sudden heart failure may cause

    _____.

19. Cystitis is an inflammation of the bladder that may be caused by a _____ infection.

20. Loss of voluntary control over urination is known as _____.

21. _____ are crystals of calcium phosphate.

9

Regulators of Body Functions

The two main communication systems of the body are the endocrine system, which acts as a chemical messenger, and the nervous system, which sends nerve impulses to all of the body structures. The endocrine system is relatively slow in its processes of hormonal regulation when compared to neural regulation and its more rapid pace.

The Endocrine System

Each endocrine gland has specific functions to perform within the body, any disturbance of which may cause changes in the body's appearance and/or functioning. Thus, the endocrine glands could be called the regulators of body functions.

A gland is any organ that produces a secretion. The endocrine glands are ductless, organized groups of tissues that use materials from the blood or lymph to make hormones. Hormones are secreted directly into the bloodstream as the blood circulates through the gland and are then transported to areas of the body, where they have an influence on various cells, tissues, and organs.

The six important endocrine glands or groups of glands in the body are the pituitary gland, located at the base of the brain; the thyroid gland, located in the neck; the parathyroid glands (in the region of the thyroid gland); the pancreas, which lies behind the stomach; the two adrenal glands, located over each kidney; and the gonads, or sex glands, meaning the ovaries in the female and the testes in the male. (See Figure 9–1.)

The Pituitary Gland

The pituitary gland, or hypophysis, is called the "master gland" because it secretes several hormones into the bloodstream that affect other endocrine glands and help to maintain proper body functioning.

The pituitary gland is responsible for the growth of the long bones (which controls the height of an individual). It influences the organs of reproduction, maintains the water balance in the body, and affects the use of starch and sugar. (See Table 9–1.)

Other Glands

The **thyroid (THEYE-royd)** gland regulates body metabolism and is located on either side of the larynx, where it maintains a rich blood supply. The thyroid gland secretes three hormones: thyroxine and triiodothyronine, both iodine-bearing derivatives of the amino-acid tyrosine, which serve to regulate the system; and calcitonin, which controls the calcium ion concentration in the body by maintaining the proper calcium

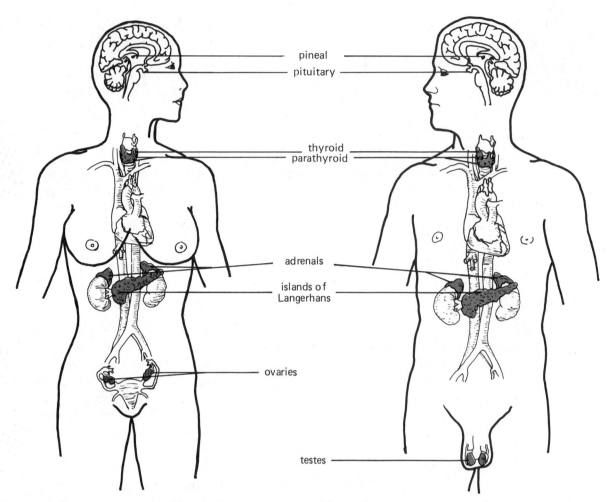

Figure 9–1   Location of the endocrine glands

level in the bloodstream. Calcium is an essential body mineral which is necessary for blood clotting, holding cells together, and neuromuscular functions.

The **thymus (THEYE-mus)** gland serves as an endocrine gland and as a lymphatic organ until it begins to disappear during puberty. The hormones secreted by the thymus help stimulate the lymphoid cells, which are responsible for the production of antibodies against certain diseases.

The **adrenal (ah-DREE-nul)** glands, located on top of each kidney, secrete hormones that are very effective as anti-inflammatory drugs. They also produce **corticoids,** which speed up the reabsorption of sodium into the blood circulation, increase the excretion of potassium from the blood, accelerate the reabsorption of water by the kidneys, increase the amount of glucose in the blood, increase cardiac output and venous return, and raise the systolic blood pressure.

The **gonads,** or sex glands, are responsible for fertility and reproduction in both sexes.

The **pancreas (PAN-kree-us)** is an organ with glandular cells that regulate the production of pancreatic juice and inlet cells that secrete the hormone insulin. The pancreas is considered to be a gland of both internal and external secretions. Insulin

Table 9-1   Pituitary Hormones and Their Known Functions

PITUITARY HORMONE	KNOWN FUNCTION
Anterior Lobe	
TSH — Thyroid-Stimulating Hormone (Thyrotropin)	Stimulates the growth and the secretion of the thyroid gland
ACTH — Adrenocorticotrophic Hormone	Stimulates the growth and the secretion of the adrenal cortex
FSH — Follicle-Stimulating Hormone	Stimulates growth of new graafian (ovarian) follicle and secretion of estrogen by follicle cells in the female and the production of sperm in the male
LH — Luteinizing Hormone (female)	Stimulates ovulation and formation of the corpus luteum
ICSH — Interstitial Cell-Stimulating Hormone (male)	Stimulates testosterone secretion
LTH — Lactogenic Hormone (Prolactin or luteotropin)	Stimulates secretion of milk and influences maternal behavior
GH — Growth Hormone (Somatotropin, STH)	Accelerates body growth
Posterior Lobe	
VASOPRESSIN (Antidiuretic Hormone, ADH)	Maintains water balance by reducing urinary output. It acts on kidney tubules to reabsorb water into the blood more quickly
OXYTOCIN	Promotes milk ejection and causes contraction of the smooth muscles of the uterus

promotes the utilization of glucose in the cells, where it also promotes fatty acid transport and fat deposition, promotes amino acid transport into the cells and facilitates protein synthesis. The lack of insulin secretion causes diabetes mellitus.

Disorders of the Endocrine System

Endocrine disturbances may be caused by a disease of the gland itself, infections in other parts of the body, or through dietary deficiencies. Most disorders are the result of either hyperactivity of the gland, causing an oversecretion of hormones, or hypoactivity of the gland, resulting in undersecretion. Because the thyroid gland controls metabolic activity, any disorder that affects the thyroid will affect other structures as well.

Hyperthyroidism is overactivity of the thyroid gland which leads to enlargement of the gland and an increase in the basal metabolic rate. Individuals with hyperthyroidism may consume a large amount of food and still suffer loss of weight and body fat. They may also suffer from increased blood pressure and heart rate, tremors, perspiration, irritability, and elevated blood sugar. Treatment of hyperthyroidism includes partial or total removal of the thyroid and the administration of drugs.

Hypothyroidism is the result of the thyroid failing to secrete sufficient thyroxine and is manifested by a low metabolic rate and decelerated body processes. Hypothyroidism may develop at any time from early infancy to adulthood. The intensity and

ability to treat hypothyroidism will depend on when the disorder occurs and how mature the system is to begin with. Some variations of the disorder may be treated with drugs to restore a normal metabolism; however, when hypothyroidism affects infants or children, in most cases, normal development cannot be completely restored.

Pituitary Disorders

The pituitary gland is mainly involved in growth function, and because it also works as the master gland, it influences other activities as well.

Gigantism is the result of hypersecretion of the pituitary growth hormone which causes an overgrowth of the long bones during preadolescence, leading to excessive height. If a pituitary tumor is responsible for the hypersecretion of growth hormones, surgery or x-ray therapy may provide some relief.

Hypofunctioning of the pituitary gland during childhood leads to pituitary dwarfism due to an inadequate production of growth hormones. Treatment involves early detection and injections of human growth hormones.

Adrenal Disorders

Overactivity of the adrenal gland may result in virilism, the development of male secondary sex characteristics in a woman such as facial hair, broad shoulders, and small breasts. Hypoactivity of the gland may lead to Addison's disease, which exhibits the following symptoms: excessive pigmentation which results in a characteristic "bronzing" of the skin, carbohydrate imbalances due to decreased levels of blood glucose, a severe blood pressure drop, muscular weakness and fatigue, gastrointestinal malfunctions, retention of water in the body tissues, and a severe drop of sodium in blood and tissue fluids, causing a serious imbalance of electrolytes.

NOTE: Electrolytes are electrically charged particles that help determine fluid and acid-base balances in the body.

Gonad disorders include cysts, tumors, and menstruation abnormalities.

Pancreatic disorders may cause diabetes mellitus, a decreased secretion of insulin that disturbs carbohydrate metabolism in the system, or diabetes insipidus, which is due to a lack of the antidiuretic hormone.

9

Fill in the Blank

1. Endocrine glands have _____ functions to perform.

2. A _____ is any organ that produces a secretion.

3. Endocrine glands are _____ glands.

4. Materials from the blood or lymph are used by the endocrine glands to make _____

5. Hormones are secreted _____ into the bloodstream.

6. The hypophysis is also known as the _____ gland.

7. The pituitary gland is called the _____ gland.

8. _____ gland secretions affect other endocrine glands.

9. Growth of the long bones is dependent on the _____ gland.

10. The pituitary gland affects the body's use of _____ and _____.

11. The thyroid gland regulates body _____.

12. Proper calcium levels in the body are maintained by the _____ gland.

13. Calcium is necessary for _____.

14. The thymus gland _____ during puberty.

15. Hormones secreted by the adrenal glands are effective as _____ drugs.

16. _____ are important hormones secreted by the adrenal glands.

17. The gonads are responsible for _____ and _____.

18. The pancreas is a gland that produces both _____ and _____ secretions.

19. _____ promotes the utilization of glucose in the cells.

20. _____ may be caused by disease of the gland, infections in other parts of the body, or dietary deficiencies.

21. Most endocrine disorders are due to _____ or _____ of the gland.

22. Any disorder that affects the _____ gland will affect other structures.

23. _____ leads to glandular enlargement and and increased metabolic rate.

24. An _____ thyroid results in hypothyroidism.

25. Gigantism is the result of hypersecretion by the _____ gland.

26. Hypofunctioning of the pituitary gland during childhood may result in _____.

27. Adrenal gland overactivity in women may lead to the development of _____ secondary sex characteristics.

28. Electrically charged particles that determine fluid and acid-base balances in the body are known as _____.

29. _____ disorders may cause diabetes mellitus.

Matching

30–35. Identify the location of each of the following endocrine glands.

30. _____ Pituitary   a. ovaries (female), testes (male)

31. _____ Thyroid   b. in the region of the thyroid

32. _____ Parathyroid   c. at the base of the brain

33. _____ Pancreas   d. located in the neck

34. _____ Adrenal glands   e. located behind the stomach

35. _____ Gonads   f. located over each kidney

10 The Nervous System

Communications within the nervous system occur at a much more rapid pace than the chemical messages within the endocrine system. The nervous system provides tools by which humans reason, learn, remember, and take part in distinctly human activities.

The nervous system is the most highly organized system of the body and consists of the brain, spinal cord, and nerves. The nerve cell, or **neuron (NYU-ron)**, is constructed to carry out its function of communication. All healthy neurons possess the ability to react when stimulated and the ability to pass on the nerve impulse thus generated to other neurons. These characteristic abilities are known as irritability and conductivity, respectively.

The three types of neurons are **sensory**, which emerge from the skin or sense organs to send impulses toward the spinal cord and brain; **motor**, which carry messages from the brain and spinal cord to muscles and glands; and **connecting**, which carry impulses from one neuron to another. (See Figure 10–1).

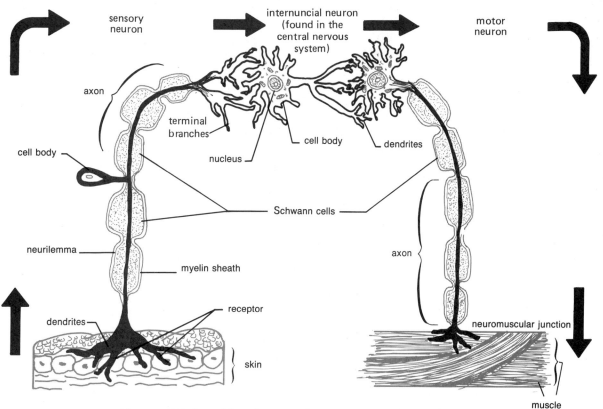

Figure 10–1   Classification of neurons according to function

The nervous system is divided into three divisions. The **central nervous system** consists of the brain and spinal cord; the **peripheral (per-IH-fer-al) nervous system** is made up of 12 pairs of cranial nerves and 31 pairs of spinal nerves; and the **autonomic** nervous system consists of peripheral nerves and ganglia that carry impulses to involuntary muscles and glands.

Decision and action involve the central and peripheral nervous systems. The autonomic nervous system supplies heart muscle, smooth muscle, and secretory glands with involuntary nervous impulses as needed for function.

The Central Nervous System

The adult human brain is a highly developed, intricate mass of nervous tissue that is protected by the bony cranial cavity and three layers of membranous material. Within the brain are four lined cavities (cerebral ventricles) that are filled with cerebrospinal fluid which acts as a liquid shock absorber for the brain and spinal cord, transports nutrients to the brain cells, and removes waste products from the brain cells.

The brain is divided into three parts: the **cerebrum (se-REE-brum)**, the **cerebellum (seh-reh-BEL-um)**, and the **brain stem**.

The cerebrum is the largest part of the brain, occupying the whole upper portion of the skull and weighing about two pounds. It is divided into two hemispheres, right and left, which are further divided into the **frontal**, **parietal (pah-re-AY-tal)**, **occipital (ok-SI-pi-tal)**, and **temporal** lobes. These lobes, whose names correspond to the adjacent cranial bones, control different types of functions. (See Figure 10–2.)

The frontal lobe control voluntary motor functions and speech. Cells in the right hemisphere of the lobe activate voluntary movements in the left side of the body, and the left hemisphere controls voluntary movements on the right side.

The parietal lobe receives and interprets nerve impulses from the sensory receptors

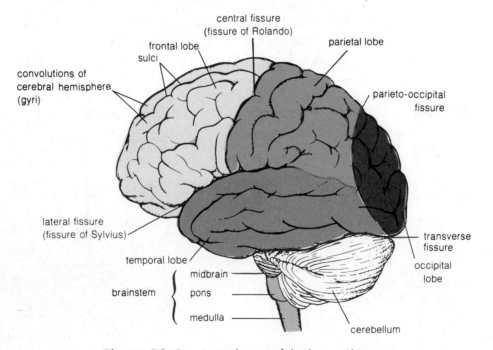

Figure 10–2   Lateral view of the human brain

for pain, touch, heat, cold, and pressure, and also helps in the determination of distances, sizes, and shapes.

The occipital lobe contains the visual area, which controls eyesight.

The upper part of the temporal lobe contains the auditory (hearing) area, while the lower (anterior) part contains the olfactory (smell) area.

The **cerebral cortex** also controls conscious thought, judgment, reasoning, memory, and will power.

Between the cerebrum and the midbrain are located two major structures—the **thalamus** and the **hypothalamus**. The thalamus acts as a relay station for incoming and outgoing nerve impulses as it receives direct and/or indirect nerve impulses from various sense organs of the body (with the exception of olfactory sensations), which are then relayed to the cerebral cortex. The thalamus also receives nerve impulses from other areas of the brain.

The hypothalamus lies below the thalamus and performs eight vital functions: autonomic nervous control (the regulation of the parasympathetic and sympathetic nervous systems); cardiovascular control, which controls blood pressure and heartbeat; temperature control; appetite control; water balance; gastrointestinal control; emotional state; and sleep control.

The **cerebellum** is located behind the pons and below the cerebrum and controls all body functions that involve skeletal muscles. Maintenance of balance and muscle tone and the coordination of secretory movements are the principal functions of the cerebellum. Injury to the cerebellum may result in impaired motor performance.

The **brain stem** is a three-part structure that includes the **midbrain, pons,** and **medulla (meh-DOO-lah).** The pons acts as a two-way pathway for nerve impulses between the cerebrum, cerebellum, and other areas of the nervous system and contains a respiration control center. The midbrain regulates sleep and wakefulness and controls moods via body chemicals that act on receptors in the midbrain. The medulla serves as a passageway for nerve impulses between the brain and the spinal cord, slows the heartbeat via the cardiac inhibitory center, controls the rate and depth of respiration, and causes the dilation and constriction of blood vessels, thereby affecting blood pressure.

The spinal cord functions as a **reflex center** and as a pathway to and from the brain. Connections that are made between incoming and outgoing nerve fibers provide the basis for reflex action. (See Table 10–1.)

The Reflex Act

The reflex act is unconscious and involuntary, the simplest type of nerve response. Blinking the eye, removing a finger from a hot object, the secretion of saliva at the sight or smell of food, and the movements of the heart, stomach, and intestines are examples of reflex actions. Every reflex act is preceded by a stimulus, which may be any change in the environment. Sound waves, light waves, heat energy, and odors are examples of stimuli that are picked up by special receptors, such as the retina of the eye (for light), the inner ear (for sound), and structures within the skin (for heat, cold, pain, and pressure). The reaction to a stimulus is called a response and may be in the form of movement, as with muscles, or secretion, as in glands.

Table 10–1 Classification of Cranial Nerves

Number–Name	Type	Function
1st Olfactory	Sensory	Controls the sense of smell
2nd Optic	Sensory	Controls the sense of sight
3rd Oculomotor	Motor	Controls the motion of the eye
4th Trochlear	Motor	Controls upward and downward motion of the eye
5th Trifacial	Sensory–Motor	Controls the sensations of the face, tongue and teeth
6th Abducent	Motor	Controls the motion of the eye
7th Facial	Sensory–Motor	Controls the motion of the face, scalp, neck, ear, palate and tongue
8th Auditory	Sensory	Controls the sense of hearing
9th Glossopharyngeal	Sensory–Motor	Controls the sense of taste
10th Vagus	Sensory–Motor	Sensory nerve of stomach, motor nerve of voice and heart
11th Accessory	Motor	Controls the motion of the neck muscles
12th Hypoglossal	Motor	Controls the motion of the tongue

Disorders of the Nervous System

Chorea (KOH-REE-ah) (St. Vitus' Dance) is a nervous system disorder that frequently appears following a streptococcal infection. It is characterized by involuntary muscular twisting and writhing movements of the arms, face, and legs. Treatment includes rest, nourishing food, and the avoidance of excitement of any kind.

Shingles (herpes zoster) is an acute viral nerve infection that is characterized by a one-sided inflammation of cutaneous nerves and which may spread to other nerves. Symptoms include painful vesicular eruptions of the skin and mucous membranes along the inflamed nerve route. Shingles often afflicts elderly or debilitated individuals.

Neuralgia (noo-RAL-jah) is a sudden, severe pain along the pathway of a nerve which may be treated with analgesics and/or narcotics.

Poliomyelitis (POH-lee-oh-meye-eh-LEYE-tis) ("polio" or infantile paralysis) is an infectious viral disease of the nerve pathways in the spinal cord that results in muscles becoming paralyzed. Death may also result. Vaccines are available to protect against polio, and all children should be immunized.

Encephalitis is a viral disease that produces inflammation of the brain. It may be caused by various organisms, certain chemical substances, or the bite of a mosquito that is carrying the virus. Although there are many forms of encephalitis, they all exhibit the following symptoms: fever, lethargy, extreme weakness, and visual disturbances. No adequate prevention methods have been developed as yet.

Cerebral palsy is a disorder of voluntary muscle action due to brian damage that may have been the result of birth injuries, intercranial hemorrhage, or infections such as encephalitis.

Convulsions are characterized by violent muscle contractions (brought on by abnormal nerve signals from the brain) as a result of rapid high fever, a calcium imbalance, or a brain tumor.

Acute bacterial **meningitis** is an inflammation of the membranes of the spinal cord or brain and may be caused by various organisms, such as tuberculosis or pneumonia. Epidemics of this disease occur frequently in close-living groups such as students in college dormitories and armed forces groups. Symptoms may include headache, fever, nasal secretions, sore throat, neck and back pain, loss of mental alertness, and rashes. Treatment may include immune serum injections, chemotherapy, and antibiotics, although limitations exist with all treatments.

Epilepsy is a disorder of the brain characterized by excessive and recurring electrical discharges from neurons and may lead to hallucinations, seizures, and unconsciousness. Most epileptic individuals can lead normal lives with regular medication.

Disorders of the Sense Organs

Ear Disorders

Otitis media is an infection of the middle ear that usually causes an earache, especially as a complication of a cold in children. Treatment includes the use of antibiotics.

Tinnitus (tih-NEYE-tis) is the sensation of ringing or buzzing in the ear and may be caused by impacted ear wax, otitis media, blockage of normal blood supply, or as a side effect of certain drugs, such as salicylates (painkillers) and quinine.

Cauliflower ear is a disfiguring condition that develops from hematomas that become calcified. It is commonly seen in boxers and wrestlers.

Eye Disorders

Conjunctivitis is a potentially contagious inflammation of the membranes in front of the eye which causes redness, pain, and a discharge of mucus. Conjunctivitis should be treated promptly by a physician. Treatments may include eye ointments or washes that contain weak solutions of isotonic saline and/or boric acid.

A **sty** is an abscess at the base of an eyelash that is due to the inflammation of a sebaceous gland of the eyelid. Nonirritating antibiotics are used for treatment.

Glaucoma is a condition in which the watery fluid of the eye does not circulate properly. This in turn causes increased pressure within the eyeball. If left untreated, glaucoma leads to blindness because it damages the retina and the optic nerve. With early detection and treatment, however, total blindness may be avoided, through the use of drugs that constrict the pupil, thus lowering eyeball pressure.

A **cataract** is characterized by a loss in transparency of the lens of the eye. Since light cannot pass through the cloudy lens, the person cannot see and may require surgery to correct the condition.

> *For the professional performing any type of massage, it is important to know that there are two types of effects of massage which may occur separately or together. These are the reflex effects and mechanical effects of massage.*

NOTE: A reflex is a point that is distant to the affected area yet when stimulated, has an effect on that area.

Gentle stimulation (such as effleurage) of the sensory nerve endings in the skin results in reflex effects which occur either locally or in other parts of the body. Both reflex and mechanical effects are experienced when direct pressure is applied to the muscles, blood and lymph vessels, or any internal structure.

The effects of massage on the nervous system depend on the direct and reflex action of the nerves being stimulated. Invigorating effects may be experienced by the entire nervous system.

Review

Fill in the Blank

1. The main communication systems of the body are the _____ system and the _____ system.

2. The nervous system consists of the _____, _____, and _____.

3. The function of neurons is to _____.

4. The three types of neurons, or nerves, are _____, _____, and _____.

5. _____ nerves emerge from the skin or sense organs.

6. The type of nerves that send impulses to the spinal cord and the brain are _____ nerves.

7. _____ nerves carry messages from the brain and spinal cord to muscles and glands.

8. Connecting nerves carry impulses from one _____ to another.

9. There are _____ divisions in the nervous system.

10. The autonomic nervous system carries impulses to _____ muscles and _____.

11. The central and peripheral nervous systems are involved in _____ making and _____.

12. The brain consists of a mass of _____ tissue.

13. Cerebrospinal fluid performs three important functions. They are:

    a. _____

    b. _____

    c. _____

14. The three parts of the brain are the: _____, _____, and the _____.

15. The largest part of the brain is the _____.

16. The cerebrum is divided into _____ hemispheres.

17. Each hemisphere is divided into _____ lobes.

18. The lobes control different types of _____.

19. Voluntary motor functions and speech are controlled by the _____ lobe.

20. The _____ lobe receives and interprets nerve impulses from sensory receptors.

21. The visual area is located in the _____ lobe.

22. The _____ lobe contains the auditory and olfactory areas.

23. The cerebral cortex controls the following abilities:

   a. _____   b. _____   c. _____

   d. _____   e. _____

24. The _____ is involved with incoming and outgoing nerve impulses.

25. Eight vital functions that the hypothalamus performs are:

   a. _____   b. _____

   c. _____   d. _____

   e. _____   f. _____

   g. _____   h. _____

26. The _____ controls all body functions that involve skeletal muscles.

27. Injury to the cerebellum may result in _____ motor performance.

28. The brainstem consists of the _____, the _____ and the _____.

29. The pons contains a _____ control center.

30. A two-way pathway for nerve impulses between the cerebrum, the cerebellum and other areas of the nervous system is located in the _____.

31. Body chemicals act on receptors in the _____.

32. The midbrain regulates _____ and controls _____.

33. Nerve impulses between the brain and the spinal cord pass through the _____.

34. The _____ affects blood pressure.

35. The spinal cord serves as a _____ center.

36. The _____ is the simplest type of nerve response.

37. Every reflex act is preceded by a _____.

38. _____ may follow a streptococcal infection.

39. Another name for shingles is _____.

40. Shingles is an acute _____ nerve infection.

41. Polio is an _____ viral disease.

42. One viral disease that affects the brain is known as _____.

43. _____ may be the result of rapid rising, high fever, calcium imbalance, or a brain tumor.

44. An inflammation of the membranes of the spinal cord or brain is called acute bacterial

    _____.

45. _____ is a disorder of the brain that involves electrical discharges.

46. An infection of the middle ear that usually causes an earache is known as _____ media.

47. _____ is the sensation of ringing or buzzing in the ears.

48. _____ is a potentially contagious inflammation of the eye membranes.

49. An inflammation of a sebaceous gland in the eyelid that results in an abscess is called a

    _____.

50. _____ is the result of the watery fluids in the eye not circulating properly.

51. A lack of transparency of the lens of the eye is a characteristic of a _____.

Matching

52–54 Identify the following components with the corresponding nervous system division.

	System	Components
52. _____	Central nervous	a. 12 pairs of cranial nerves and 31 pairs of spinal nerves
53. _____	Peripheral nervous	b. Peripheral nerves and ganglia
54. _____	Autonomic	c. Brain and spinal cord

Bibliography

Balch, James S., M.D., and Phyllis A. Balch, C.N.C. *Prescription for Nutritional Healing.* Garden City Park, N.Y.: Avery Publishing Group, Inc., 1990.

Beck, Mark. *The Theory and Practice of Therapeutic Massage.* Edited by Bobbi Ray Madry. Albany, N.Y.: Milady Publishing Company, 1989.

Burke, Shirley R. *Human Anatomy and Physiology in Health and Disease.* Albany, N.Y.: Delmar Publishers Inc., 1992.

Fong, Elizabeth, Elvira B. Ferris, and Esther G. Skelley. *Body Structures and Functions.* Albany, N.Y.: Delmar Publishers Inc., 1989.

Gerson, Joel. *Standard Textbook for Professional Estheticians.* Albany, N.Y.: Milady Publishing Company, 1989.

Gior, Fino. *Modern Electrology.* Albany, N.Y.: Milady Publishing Company, 1987.

Pourit, A. H. *Hair Structure and Chemistry Simplified.* Albany, N.Y.: Milady Publishing Company, 1990.

Scali-Sheahan, Maura T. *Milady's Standard Textbook of Professional Barber-Styling.* Albany, N.Y.: Milady Publishing Company, 1993.

Glossary/Index

NOTE: bold type headings include definitions

A

Abduction, is the movement of an extremity away from the midline, 61

Acids, are substances that, when dissolved in water, will ionize into positively charged hydrogen ions and negatively charged ions of some other element, 9

Acquired immune deficiency syndrome (AIDS), 111–13

Acquired immunity, is a reaction that occurs as a result of exposure to invaders of the body and is developed over the span of a lifetime, 108

Active acquired immunity, is the result of having been inoculated with the appropriate vaccine, antigen, or toxoid, 108

Active transport, the molecules move across the cell membrane via a carrier molecule which picks up a molecule on the outside of the cell membrane and then carries it back within the cell membrane, 14

Acute bacterial meningitis, is an inflammation of the membranes of the spinal cord or brain and may be caused by various organisms, such as tuberculosis or pneumonia, 167

Acute kidney failure, may be the result of shock, injury, bleeding, poisoning, or sudden heart failure, 152–53

Acute rheumatic heart disease, is an infection of the membrane lining the heart, most often caused by streptococci bacteria, that alters heart tissue and affects the valves, causing heart damage, 109

Adam's apple, one of the nine fibrocartilaginous plates which make up the larynx, 122

Addison's disease, results from hypoactivity of the adrenal gland, 160

Adduction, is movement toward the midline, 61

Adrenal glands, are located on top of each kidney, secrete hormones that are very effective as anti–inflammatory drugs, 158
disorders of, 160

Agglutinin, a blood protein found in the plasma, 107

Agglutinogen, a blood protein which determines blood type, 107

AIDS, 111–13

Alimentary canal, 131, 132

Alveoli, 124

Amino acids, 8
digestion and, 135
free, hold the moisture within the cortex at the desirable level of 10 percent, 49

Amphiarthroses, are partially movable joints that have cartilage between their particular surfaces, 61

Anagen stage, keratin formation and, 48–50

Anatomy, is the study of the shape and structure of an organism's body and the relationship of one body part to another, 1
study of, 1–2
terms related to, 2

Anemia, is a deficiency in the number of red blood cells and/or the ratio percentile of hemoglobin in the blood resulting from a large or chronic loss of blood, 110

Angina pectoris, is a sudden, severe chest pain that occurs when the heart does not receive enough oxygen and is usually brought on by emotional stress or physical exertion, 110

Angiology, the study of the circulatory system, 1

Ankle, contains 7 tarsal bones, which provide a connection between the foot and leg bones, 68

Ankylosis, the abnormal immobility and consolidation of a joint as a result of the bones having fused solid, 69

Anorexia nervosa, 143

Anterior, front, 2

Aorta, is the largest artery in the body and forms an arch, consisting of three branches: the brachycephalic, the left common carotid, and the left subclavian arteries, 101

Aortic semilunar valve, permits the blood to pass from the left ventricle into the aorta, 99

Apnea, is the temporary cessation of respiratory movements, 126

Apocrine glands, empty into the canal of the

follicle at the point above the sebaceous duct in the armpit, 27

Appendicitis, is inflammation of the veriform appendix, 144

Appendicular skeleton, includes the 126 bones of the upper and lower extremities, which include the body structures of the shoulder girdle, arms, hands, pelvic girdle, upper legs, lower legs, ankles, and feet, 66–68

Arm, bone structure of, 64–65

Arrhythmia, is any change from the normal, synchronized rhythm of the heart action, 110

Arteriosclerosis, is the thickening of the walls of the arteries, 110

Arthritis, an inflammatory condition of one or more joints, accompanied by pain and, often, changes in bone position, 69

Arthrology, study of the joints, 1

Asthma, is a respiratory disorder that may be triggered by emotional stress or the breathing of irritants, 127

Atrial fibrillation, is a condition in which the atria are never completely emptied of blood and their walls quiver instead of performing the usual contraction, 110

Atrioventricular valves, permit the blood to flow in only one direction, prohibiting it from flowing backward into the chambers, 98

Atrophic gastritis, is a chronic form in which the membrane has atrophied, 143

Auricles, upper chambers of the heart, 98

Autonomic nervous system, consists of peripheral nerves and ganglia that carry impulses to involuntary muscles and glands, 164

Axial skeleton, 63–66

B

Bacteria, skin and, 28

Base, or alkali is a substance that, when dissolved in water, ionizes into negatively charged hydroxide ions and positively charged ions of a metal, 9

Blood, 104–7
is a transporting fluid of the body that carries nutrients from the digestive tract to the cells, oxygen from the lungs to the cells, waste products from the cells to various organs for excretion, and hormones from secreting cells to other parts of the body, 104–5
cells, 104
the solid components of blood, 96
red, contain the red pigment hemoglobin,

which is composed of protein and iron. Hemoglobin is vital to the function of the red blood cell as it helps transport oxygen to the tissues and carbon dioxide away from them, 106
white, help protect the body against infection and injury by surrounding and digesting or destroying bacteria, by the synthesis of antibody molecules, by "cleaning up" cellular remains at inflammation sites, and by walling off infected areas, 106
circulation of, 97
function/path of, 100–103
compositional changes of, 98
disorders of, 110–11
functions of, 95–97
plasma, 105–6
the liquid portion of blood that suspends blood cells, transports them throughout the body, bring nutrients to the cells, and carries away metabolic waste products to the excretory organs, 96, 105
platelets, are the smallest solid components of blood and function in the initial blood–clotting process by producing adhesive structures that stick to collagen fibers in a wound to stop the bleeding, 106
pressure, 103–4
proteins, 105–6
RH factor, 109
types, is determined by the presence or absence of a blood protein called agglutinogen, on the surface of the red blood cell, 107
vessels, disorders of, 110

Body
cavities of, 2, 4, 5
divisions of, 3
systems, 22

Bones
disorders/injuries of, 69–70
structure/formation of, 61–63
types of, 59

Bradycardia, is an abnormally slow heartbeat (less than 60 beats per minute), 110

Brain, is a highly developed, intricate mass of nervous tissue that is protected by the bony cranial cavity and three layers of membranous material, 164
lateral view of, 164
stem, is a three–part structure that includes the midbrain, pons, and medulla, 165

Breathing, mechanics of, 125–26

Bronchi, 124

Bronchioles, 124

Bronchitis, is an inflammation of the mucous membrane of the trachea and the bronchial tubes, 127

Bunion, a swelling of the bursa of the foot,

usually of the joint in the big toe, which then becomes adducted, 70

Burns, tissue repair and, 23

Bursitis, an acute inflammation of the synovial bursa, which cushions a joint during motion, 70

C

Cancer, lungs, is a malignant tumor which often forms in the bronchial epithelium and can be difficult to detect since the apparent symptoms are few, 127

Cancer, massage and, 88

Carbohydrates, are compounds composed of the elements carbon, hydrogen, and, oxygen, 8
  digestion and, 135

Cardiac muscle tissue, makes up the wall of the heart, with an inner lining of smooth tissue called the endocardium, 98

Catagen phase, keratin formation and, 51

Cataract, is characterized by a loss in transparency of the lens of the eye, 167

Caudal
  lower or below another, 2
  tail end of body (refers to direction), 2

Cauliflower ear, is a disfiguring condition that develops from hematomas that become calcified. It is commonly seen in boxers and wrestlers, 167

Cavities, body, 2, 4, 5

Cell, 10–15
  is the basic unit of structure and function of all living things, 10
  membrane
    material movement across, 13–15
    separates the cell's cytoplasm from its external environment and from neighboring cells, 10
  structure of, 12

Cellular respiration, is a chemical process within the cells by which oxygen is used to release energy that is stored in nutrient molecules, such as glucose, 122

Central nervous system, 164–65
  consists of the brain and spinal cord, 164

Cerebellum, maintenance of balance and muscle tone and the coordination of secretory movements are the principal functions of the cerebellum, 165

Cerebral cortex, controls conscious thought, judgment, reasoning, memory, and will power, 165

Cerebral palsy, is a disorder of voluntary muscle action due to brain damage that may have been the result of birth injuries, intracranial hemorrhage, or infections such as encephalitis, 166

Cerebrum, is the largest part of the brain, occupying the whole upper portion of the skull and weighing about two pounds, 164

Chemistry, 5–10
  is the study of the structure of matter—the composition of substances, their properties, and their chemical reactions and synthesis, 5
  compounds, 7–9
  elements and, 5–7

Cholesterol, is a common animal fat that is found in animal cell membranes, 135

Chorea, is a nervous system disorder that frequently appears following a streptococcal infection, 166

Circulatory system, 95
  carries oxygen and nourishment to cells of body; carries waste from cells; body defense, 21
  disorders of
    blood, 110
    blood vessels, 110
    heart, 109–10

Cirrhosis, is a chronic and progressive inflammation of the liver commonly caused by excessive alcohol consumption, 144

Closed fracture, the bone is broken but the broken ends do not pierce the skin, 69

Clubfoot, a congenital malformation that may involve one or both feet, 70

Colitis, is a condition in which the colon becomes inflamed and is accompanied by excessive mucus secretions, 144

Comminuted fracture, the bone is splintered or broken into many pieces that can become embedded in the surrounding tissue, 69

Comparative anatomy, is the study of the different body parts and organs of humans with regard to the similarities and differences to other species in the animal kingdom, 1

Compounds, 7–9
  are elements combined together in a definite proportion by weight, 7

Congenital heart disease, is a condition that is present at birth in which the heart did not develop properly during in the uterus, 110

Congestive heart failure, is similar to heart failure, with the addition of swelling in the lower extremities. Blood backs up into the lung vessels and fluid extends into the air passages, 110

Conjunctivitis, is a potentially contagious inflammation of the membranes in front of the eye which caused redness, pain, and a discharge of mucus, 167

Connecting neurons, carry impulses from one neuron to another, 163

Connective tissue, 19–21

Convulsions, are characterized by violent muscle contractions as a result of rapid high fever, a calcium imbalance, or a brain tumor, 166

Cooley's anemia, is a chronic blood disease, inherited from both parents, that causes red blood cells to form in an abnormal shape, 111

Coronary occlusion, is a condition in which the heart does not receive enough blood due to blockage in a coronary artery, 110

Cortex, is a complicated formation of millions of parallel fibers of hard keratin, referred to as polypeptide chains, that twist around one another in a rope fashion, 43-45
   hair
      bonds of, 48
      cuticle and, 45

Corticoids, speed up reabsorption of sodium into blood circulation, increase excretion of potassium, accelerate reabsorption of water by the kidneys, increase the amount of glucose in the blood, increase cardiac output and venous return, raise systolic blood pressure, 158

Cranial, head end of the body (refers to direction), 2

Cranial nerves, classification of, 166

Cuticle, is the outside layer of the hair shaft. It consists of hard, flattened scales that overlap one another with an average thickness of seven scales, 42–43
   cortex and, 45
   keratinization of, 50
   nail, is the overlapping skin around the nail, 27

Cystine bonds, join the chains of peptide bonds together horizontally, like rungs of a ladder, 48

Cystitis, is an inflammation of the mucous membrane lining of the urinary bladder that has spread to the bladder, 153

Cytology, the study of the structure, function, and development of cells that make up the different body parts, 1

Cytoplasm, is a sticky, semifluid substance found between nucleus and the cell membrane, 10

D

Dermatology, study of the integumentary system (skin, hair & nails), 1

Dermis, is the thicker, inner layer of the skin that contains matted masses of connective tissue; strong, fibrous tissue bands; elastic fibers; lymphatics; nerve endings; muscles; hair follicles; oil and sweat glands; and fat cells, 25

Developmental anatomy, studies the growth and development of a organism during its lifetime, 1

Diabetes
   insipidus, is due to a lack of the antidiuretic hormone, 160
   mellitus, is caused by a decreased secretion of insulin that disturbs carbohydrate metabolism in the system, 160

Dietary guidelines, 139, 141

Diffusion, 13–14
   is a physical, passive process whereby molecules of gases, liquids, or solid particles disperse themselves evenly through a medium, 13

Digestion, is the changing of complex insoluble food molecules into simple soluble molecules so they can be transported by the blood to the cells and be absorbed through the cell membranes, 133

Digestive system, consists of the alimentary canal and accessory digestive organs, 133
   It also prepares food for absorption and use by body cells through modification of chemical and physical states, 21
   disorders of, 143–44
   eating disorders and, 142–43
   nutrients and, 135–36

Digestive tract, consists of the mouth, throat, esophagus, stomach, small intestines, large intestines (colon), and anus, 133

Diphtheria, is a highly infectious disease that affects the upper respiratory tract and can be recognized by the formation of a grayish–white or yellow membrane on the pharynx, larynx, trachea, and/or tonsils, 127

Disaccharides, are formed by two monosaccharide molecules and are known as double sugars, 8

Dislocation, the bone is displaced from its proper position in the joint, which may result in tearing or stretching of ligaments, 69

Distal, away from the point of attachment or origin, 2

Dorsal, back, 2

Dyspnea, is difficult, labored, or painful breathing in conjunction with discomfort and breathlessness, 126

Dysuria, is difficult urination, 153

E

Ear, disorders of, 167

Eating disorders, 142–43

Eccrine glands, open directly onto the surface of the skin, where they secrete large amounts of diluted salt water when stimulated by heat or emotional stress, 27

Edema, 88

Electrolytes, act as chemical buffers in helping to maintain the acid–base balance of the blood, 106

are electrically charged particles that help determine fluid and acid–base balances in the body, 160

Elements, 5–6

Embolism, is a condition in which a foreign substance, (embolus) such as air, a blood clot, cancer of fat cells, or bacterial clumps is carried by the bloodstream until it reaches an artery that is too small for passage, 110–11

Emphysema, is a noninfectious condition in which the lungs become overinflated, with the result that breathing is made difficult, 127

Encephalitis, is a viral disease that produces inflammation of the brain, 166

End–bonds, are chemical bonds that join the amino acids in a chain, 48

Endocarditis, is an inflammation of the membrane lining, 110

Endocardium, covers the heart valves and lines the blood vessel to provide smooth transit of the flowing blood, 98

Endocrine glands, are ductless organized groups of tissues that use materials from the blood or lymph to make hormones, 157

location of, 158

Endocrine system, 157–60

manufactures hormones to regulate organ activity, 21

disorders of, 159–60

Endocrinology, study of the endocrine, or hormonal system, 2

Enteritis, is an inflammation of the intestine caused by a bacterial, viral, or protozoan infection, food poisoning, or an allergic reaction to certain food, 144

Enzymatic hydrolysis, is the changing of complex insoluble food molecules into simple soluble molecules so they can be transported by the blood to the cells and be absorbed through the cell membranes, 133

Enzymes, are chemical substances that promote chemical changes in living things

without themselves being affected by the reactions, 133

are specialized protein molecules found in all living cells and help control the various chemical reactions occurring within them, 8

help the body to control its chemical reactions, 104

Epidermis, forms the outer, protective covering of the skin, and although it does not contain blood vessels, it does have many small nerve endings, 23

Epilepsy, is a disorder of the brain characterized by excessive and recurring electrical discharges from neurons and may lead to hallucinations, seizures, and unconsciousness, 167

Epithelial tissue, 16–17

Eponychium, is the thin line of skin at the base of the nail that extends from the nail wall to the nail plate, 27

Erythrocytes, contain the red pigment hemoglobin, which is composed of protein and iron. Hemoglobin is vital to the function of the red blood cell as it helps transport oxygen to the tissues and carbon dioxide away from them, 106

Eupnea, is normal breathing, with the usual quiet inhalations and exhalations, 126

Excretory system, removes waste products of metabolism from the body, 23

disorders of, 152–53

urinary tract, 151–52

waste elimination and, 151

Exhalation, 125

Extension, means to straighten the forearm or fingers, 61

External respiration, is the exchange of oxygen and carbon dioxide between the body and the outside environment, 121

Eye, disorders of, 167

F

Face

muscles of, 84

sagittal section of, 121

Facial expression, muscles of, 77

Filtration, is the movement of solutes and water across a semipermeable membrane that results from some mechanical force such as blood pressure or gravity, 14

Flatfeet, are the result of the downward pressure of the body weight on the foot, which flattens the arches due to a weakening of the leg muscles, 86

Follicles, are small downgrowths into the dermis, 37
  origin of, 40
  structure of, 39–42
Foods
  processing of, 141–42
  protein in, 39–42
Foot, has five metatarsal bones, which are somewhat comparable to the metacarpals of the hand, 68
  dorsal view of, 68
Fractures, bone, 69
Free amino acids, hold the moisture within the cortex at the desirable level of 10 percent, 49
Free edge, is the end of the nail that extends beyond the fingertip, 26
Frontal lobe, control voluntary motor functions and speech, 164

G

Gallbladder, is the storehouse of bile for the liver, releasing it as needed for the digestion of fats, 133
Gallstones, are deposits of crystallized cholesterol that form in the gallbladder, 144
Gangrene, results when an insufficient blood supply, due to disease or injury, causes death of body tissue, 110
Gastritis, is an acute or chronic inflammation of the stomach's mucous membrane lining caused by spicy food or some drugs, 143
Gigantism, is the result of hypersecretion of the pituitary growth hormone which causes an overgrowth of the long bones, during preadolescence, leading to excessive height, 160
Gland, is any organ that produces a secretion, 157
Glaucoma, is a condition in which the watery fluid of the eye does not circulate properly. This causes increased pressure within the eye. If left untreated, glaucoma leads to blindness, 167
Gonads, are responsible for fertility and reproduction in both sexes, 158
  disorders of, 160
Gouty arthritis, is caused by a faulty uric acid metabolism and occurs more often in overweight individuals and those who regularly indulge in rich foods and alcohol, 70
Greenstick fracture, the simplest type of fracture, in which the bone is partially bent but does not completely separate, 69
Gross anatomy, is the study of large and easily observable structures of an organism, 1

H

Hair, 26
  Cortex
    is a complicated formation of millions of parallel fibers of hard keratin, referred to as polypeptide chains, that twist around one another in a rope fashion, 43–45
    bonds of, 48–49
    cuticle and, 45
  cuticle, is the outside layer of the hair shaft. It consists of hard, flattened scales that overlap one another with an average thickness of seven scales, 42–43
  follicle. See Follicles
  growth of, 46–49
  keratin, formation of, 49–51
  lanugo, 37–38
    soft, downy hair. Most of the lanugo hair is shed prior to birth except in the regions of the eyebrows, eyelids, and scalp, 37
  medulla, is the central layer of the hair. It is made up of a column of cells, either two or four rows wide, 46
  origin of, 40
  root, 41–42
  secondary, 38
    is more stiff and bristly than the lanugo hair, 37
  tertiary, 38–39
    is the long, soft hair found on the scalp, the beard and mustache of adult males, and the legs and underarms of all adults, 37
Hand, is composed of 5 metacarpal bones and 14 phalanges, 67
  bones of, view of, 67
Head, muscles, 84
  control facial expression and the act of mastication, 76
Heart, is a tough, simply constructed muscle about the size of a closed fist, measuring 5 inches long and 3 1/2 inches wide, weighing less than a pound, 98
  anterior view of, 99
  block, is the loss of ability of a damaged A–V node to carry nerve impulses, 110
  disorders of, 109–110
  failure, is the inability of the heart muscles to beat efficiently and may be caused by high blood pressure or other pathological conditions, 110
  murmurs, may indicate some functional defect in the valves of the heart, 110

structure of, 98–99

Heartburn, is a condition that results from the backflow of the highly acidic gastric juices to the lower end of the esophagus which irritates the lining, causing a burning sensations, 143

Hematoma, is a localized mass of blood found in an organ, tissue, or space as a result of injury that can cause a blood vessel to rupture, 111

Hemodialysis, is the process by which an artificial kidney machine is used to remove waste products from the kidneys, 153

Hemophilia, is a hereditary disease in which the blood clots too slowly to prevent or prolonged bleeding, 111

Hemorrhoids, are varicosities in the walls of the lower rectum and the tissues around the anus, 110

Herpes zoster, is an acute viral nerve infection that is characterized by a one–sided inflammation of cutaneous nerves and which may spread to other nerves, 166

Hiatal hernia, is a rupture that occurs when the stomach protrudes above the diaphragm through the esophagus opening, 143

High blood pressure, means excessive pressure of the blood against the walls of the arteries, 88

Histology, studies the tissues and organs making up the entire body of an organism, 1

HIV, 111–13

Hormones, help the body to control its chemical reactions, 106

Human development, 4

Human immunodeficiency virus, 111–13

Hydrogen bonds, are the most numerous bonds in the hair and help the sulphur bond keep the parallel chains of amino acids together, 48

Hyperpnea, is an increase in the depth and rate of breathing in conjunction with exaggerated respiratory movements, 126

Hypersensitivity, occurs when the body's immune system fails to protect itself against foreign material, 108

Hypertension, 103

Hyperthyroidism, is overactivity of the thyroid gland which leads to enlargement of the gland and an increase in the basal metabolic rate, 159

Hyponychium, is the part of the skin under the free edge of the nail, 27

Hypophysis, is called the "master gland" because it secretes several hormones into the bloodstream that affect other endocrine glands and help to maintain proper body functioning, 157

Hypothalamus, performs eight vital functions: autonomic nervous control; cardiovascular control; temperature control; appetite control; water balance; gastrointestinal control; emotional state; and sleep control, 165

Hypothyroidism, is the result of the thyroid failing to secrete sufficient thyroxine and is manifested by a low metabolic rate and decelerated body processes, 159–60

I

Immunity
lymphatic system, 107–9
types of, 108

Immunization, is the process of increasing an individual's resistance to a particular infection by artificial means, 108

Incontinence, occurs when an individual loses voluntary control over urination, resulting in voiding whenever the bladder fills, 153

Infantile paralysis, is an infectious viral disease of the nerve pathways in the spinal cord that results in muscles becoming paralyzed, 166

Infectious gastritis, is an acute form associated with infectious diseases, 143

Infectious hepatitis, is a viral infection of the liver caused by contaminated food or water, 144

Inferior, lower or below another, 2

Inflammation, occurs when living tissue is damaged by chemical or physical trauma or through the invasion of pathogenic bacteria. Characteristic symptoms of inflammation include redness, localized heat, swelling, and pain, 106

Inhalation, 123

Inorganic compounds, are generally compounds that do not contain the element carbon, 8

Integumentary system, helps regulate body temperature; establishes a barrier between the body and the environment; eliminates waste; synthesizes vitamin D; contains receptors for temperature, pressure, and pain, 21
appendages of, 26–28
structures of, 23–28

Internal, involving an internal organ or structure, 2

Internal respiration, involves the exchange of carbon dioxide and oxygen between cells and the surrounding lymph, and the oxidative process of energy in the cells, 122

Intestine, large, acts in absorbing water, nonpathogenic bacterial action, fecal formation, and defecation, 134

Intestine, small, begins and finishes fat digestion and completes the digestion process of carbohydrates and proteins, 133

Iron–deficiency anemia, is a condition caused by inadequate amounts of iron in the diet which may be corrected by iron supplements or foods that contain the mineral, 110

J

Joints, 59–61
  disorders/injuries of, 69–70
  motion of, 61

K

Keratin, a nonliving protein substance which acts as a waterproof covering, 23
  formation of, 49–51

Kidney stones, are microscopic crystals of calcium phosphate that clump together when stagnation of urine occurs, eventually blocking the urine flow in the ureter, 153

Kidneys, are bean–shaped organs located against the dorsal wall of the abdominal cavity and on either side of the vertebral column, 151

L

Lactic acid, muscle fatigue and, 76

Lanugo hair, 37–38
  soft, downy hair. Most of the lanugo hair is shed prior to birth except in the regions of the eyebrows, eyelids, and scalp, 37

Large intestine, acts in absorbing water, nonpathogenic bacterial action, fecal formation, and defecation, 134

Laryngitis, is an inflammation of the voice box that is often secondary to other respiratory infections, 127

Larynx, is a triangular chamber located below the pharynx that is composed of nine fibrocartilaginous plates, 122, 124

Lateral, away, or toward the side of the body, 2

Leukemia, is a condition in which there is an overproduction of white blood cells which replace the red blood cells and interfere with the transport of oxygen to the tissues, 111

Life functions, 4, 6

Lipids, are molecules containing the elements carbon, hydrogen, and oxygen, 8, 135
  digestion and, 135

Liver bile, aids in the digestion of fat, 133

Lower extremities, muscles, assist in the movement of the thigh (femur), leg, ankle, foot, and toes, 76, 78

Lumbago, a backache in the lower lumbar region of the spinal column, 70

Lungs, are two cone–shaped organs situated in the lateral chambers of the thoracic cavity, where they are separated by the mediastinum and the heart, 124
  cancer of, is a malignant tumor which often forms in the bronchial epithelium and can be difficult to detect since the apparent symptoms are few, 127

Lunula, is the light–colored half–moon shape at the base of the nail, 27

Lymph, is a straw–colored fluid composed of water, lymphocytes, granulocytes, oxygen, digested nutrients, hormones, salts, carbon dioxide, and urea, 107
  nodes, are situated either alone or grouped in various places along the lymph vessels throughout the body. Their function is to provide sites for lymphatic production and to serve as a filter for screening out harmful substances from the lymph, 108
  vessels, accompany and parallel the veins and are located in most of the tissues and organs that have blood vessels, 108

Lymphatic system
  can be considered a supplement to the circulatory system and consists of lymph, lymph nodes, lymph vessels, the spleen, the thymus gland, lymphoid tissue, and tonsils, 105, 107
  immunity and, 107–9

M

Massage
  client preparation for, 80–81
  effects of, 88–89
  movements, 81–82
  room equipment, 80
  scalp, 83, 85
    procedure, 87
  skeletal muscles involved in, 81
  varicose veins and, 103

Mastication, muscles of, 77

Matrix, the nail bed which contains nerves with lymph and blood vessels which produce nail cells and control the rate of growth of the nail, 27

Matter, can exist in one of three states or phases—solid, liquid, and gas, 5

Medial, toward the midline plane of the body, 2

Medulla, a passageway for nerve impulses between the brain and the spinal cord, slows heartbeat via cardiac inhibitory center, controls rate and depth of respiration, and causes dilation and construction of blood vessels, affecting blood pressure, 165

hair, is the central layer of the hair. It is made up of a column of cells, either two or four rows wide, 46

Melanin, pigment which gives color to the skin, 25

Melanocytes, are found within the germinativum cells and contains melanin, or skin pigment, 25

Metabolic waste products, are formed by the chemical reactions occurring to maintain homeostasis, 106

Metabolism, is the sum of all the chemical relations within a cell, including functional activities, which result in growth, repair, energy release, the use of food, and secretions, 4

Microscopic anatomy, is a branch of anatomy that is subdivided into two types—cytology and histology, 1

Midbrain, regulates sleep and wakefulness and controls moods via body chemicals that act on receptors in the midbrain, 165

Mineral salts, act as chemical buffers in helping to maintain the acid–base balance of the blood, 106

Minerals, are natural chemical elements found in the earth that, like vitamins, function as coenzymes, 136

needed for health, 140

supplements needed for assimilation of, 137

Mitosis, is the division process of cells, during which the nuclear material is distributed to each of the two new nuclei, 10

stages of, 13

Mitral bicuspid valve, allows blood flow from the left atrium to the left ventricle, 99

Molecules, are the smallest unit of a compound that still has the properties of the compound and has the ability to lead its own stable and independent existence, 7

Monosaccharides, are single or simple sugars which cannot be broken down further, such as glucose, fructose, and galactose, 8

Motion, types of, 61

Motor neuron, carries messages from the brain and spinal cord to muscles and glands, 163

Murmurs, may indicate some functional defect in the valves of the heart, 110

Muscles
atrophy of, 85–86

attachment of, 75–79

belly, is the central area or body of the muscle, 76

characteristics of, 75

face, 84

fatigue, 76

may occur from the temporary overuse of muscles, 86

head, 84

control facial expression and the act of mastication, 76, 77

hypertrophy, results from overworking or overexercising, whereby the muscles enlarge and becomes stronger, 86

insertion, is the end which is attached to a movable part and moves the most during a muscle contraction, 76

lower extremities, assist in the movement of the thigh (femur), leg, ankle, foot, and toes, 76, 78, 79

massage, 81

effects of, 88–89

neck, 84

move the head through extension, flexion, and rotation movements, 76, 77

origin, is the part of a skeletal muscle that is attached to a fixed structure or bone which moves least during muscle contraction, 76

spasms, sudden and violent contractions may be caused by the sudden overworking of a muscle or by poor circulation to the localized area, 86

stimulation of, 82

tissue, 20

tone of, is the condition of a muscle always being slightly contracted and ready to pull, 76

trunk, control breathing and the movements of the abdomen and the pelvis, 76, 78

types of, 75

upper extremities, help move the shoulder (scapula), arm (humerus), forearm, wrist, hand, and fingers, 76, 78

Muscular system, determines posture; procedures body heat; provides for movement, 21

Musculoskeletal disorders, 85–86

Myalgia, is muscular pain, 86

Myocardium, makes up the wall of the heart, with an inner lining of smooth tissue called the endocardium, 98

Myology, study of the muscular system, 2

N

Nail
   bed, is the portion of skin beneath the nail body on which the nail plates rest, 26
   body, is the main part of the nail and is attached to the skin at the tip of the finger, 26
   grooves, are slits or tracks in the nail bed at the sides of the nail on which the nail grows, 27
   mantle, is the deep fold of skin at the base of the nail where the nail root is embedded, 27
   wall, is the skin on the sides of the nail above the grooves, 27
Nails, are hard structures of keratinized plates that cover the dorsal surfaces of the last phalanges of the fingers and toes, 26
Nasal cavity, 122
Natural acquired immunity, is the result of the body producing antibodies after having had, and recovered from a particular disease, 108
Neck, muscles, move the head through extension, flexion, and rotation movements, 76, 77, 84
   sagittal section of, 121
   stiff, 86
Neoplasms, various types of tumors that can occur in bones, 70
Nerve cells, 163
Nerves, tissue, 20
Nervous system, 163–67
   communicates; controls body activity; coordinates body activity, 21
   disorders of, 166–67
Neuralgia, is a sudden, severe pain along the pathway of a nerve which may be treated with analgesics and/or narcotics, 166
Neurology, study of the nervous system, 2
Neuron, is constructed to carry out its function of communication within the nervous system, 163
Nucleic acids, are essential organic compounds containing the elements carbon, oxygen, hydrogen, nitrogen, and phosphorous, 9

O

Obesity, 142–43
Occipital lobe, of the brain, contains the visual area, which controls eyesight, 165
Open fracture, the most serious type of fracture, in which the broken bone ends pierce through the skin, forming an external wound that is subject to infection, 69
Organ system, a group of organs that act together to perform a specific and related function, 21
Organelles, cell structures, 10
Organic compounds, always contain the element carbon combined with hydrogen and elements, 8
Organs, 21
   of the body function independently with one another to form a whole, live, functioning organism, 4
Orthopnea, is difficult or labored breathing when the body is in a prone position, which may be corrected by assuming a sitting or standing position, 126
Osmosis, 15
   is the diffusion of water or any other solvent molecule through a selective permeable membrane, such as a cell membrane, 14
Ossa carpi, the wrist bone, consists of eight small bones arranged in two rows that are held together by ligaments which allow mobility and flexion, 67
Osteoarthritis, a degenerative joint disease in which the cartilage at the ends of the bones progressively wears down, the joint position, 69
Osteology, study of the skeletal system, 2
Osteoporosis, a gradual loss of bone mass in both men and women, usually caused by hormonal imbalances, 70
Otitis media, is an infection of the middle ear that usually causes an earache, especially as a complication of a cold in children, 167

P

Pancreas, is an organ with glandular cells that regulate the production of pancreatic juice and inlet cells that secrete the hormone insulin, 158–59
Papillae, ridges located at the lower edge of the stratum germinativum, 25
Papillary layer, lies directly beneath the epidermis and contains cone–shaped projections of elastic tissue (papillae) that point upward into the epidermis, 25
Parietal lobe, receives and interprets nerve impulses from the sensory receptors for pain, touch, heat, cold, and pressure, and also helps in the determination of distances, sizes, and shapes, 165
Passive acquired immunity, is acquired artificially through the injection of antibodies, which act immediately to

provide temporary protection that lasts from three to five weeks, 108

Pelvic girdle, serves as area of attachment for the bones and muscles of the leg, in addition to providing support for the soft organs of the lower abdominal region, 67

Peptic ulcers, are lesions that occur in either the stomach or the small intestines as the result of insufficient mucus secretion and an oversecretion of gastric juice, 143

Peptide bonds, are chemical bonds that join the amino acids in a chain, 48

Perionychium, is the part of the skin bordering the root and sides of the nail, 27

Peripheral nervous system, is made up of 12 pairs of cranial nerves and 31 pairs of spinal nerves, 164

Pertussis, is an infectious disease characterized by repeated coughing attacks that end in a "whooping" sound, 127

pH, is the measure of acidity (hydrogen ions) or alkalinity (hydroxide ions) of a solution, 9–10
    values, 11

Phagocytosis, is the process of the ingestion of foreign or other particles by certain cells, 15

Pharyngitis, may be the result of bacteria, viruses, or irritants, including too much smoking or speaking, and is characterized by a red, inflamed throat, painful swallowing, and extreme dryness of the throat, 127

Pharynx, 122

Phlebitis, is an inflammation of the lining of a vein accompanied by clotted blood, 88, 110

Physiology, studies the function of each body part and how these functions coordinate to form a complete living organism, 1

Physiotherapy, 79–85
    is the treatment of disease and injury by physical means, using light, heat, cold, water, electricity, massage and exercise, 79

Pituitary dwarfism, is due to an inadequate production of growth hormones, 160

Pituitary gland, is called the "master gland" because it secretes several hormones into the bloodstream that affect other endocrine glands and help to maintain proper body functioning, 157
    disorders of, 160
    hormones of, 159

Plasma. See Blood, plasma

Pneumonia, is an infection of the lung(s), usually caused by bacteria, whereby the alveoli fill up with fluid, 127

Poliomyelitis, is an infectious viral disease of the nerve pathways in the spinal cord that results in muscles becoming paralyzed, 166

Polypnea, is rapid respiration or panting due to emotional trauma or increased muscular activity, 126

Polysaccharides, are found in, or made by, living organisms and microbes and consist of glucose molecules bonded together in a chain–like fashion, 8

Pons, acts as a two–way pathway for nerve impulses between the cerebrum, cerebellum, and other areas of the nervous system and contains a respiration control center, 165

Posterior, back, 2

Potential hydrogen (pH), is the measure of acidity (hydrogen ions) or alkalinity (hydroxide ions) of a solution, 9–10
    values, 11

Pregnancy, massage and, 88

Protein
    digestion and, 135–36
    in foods, 136
    hair growth and, 46–49
    is composed of carbon, hydrogen, oxygen, nitrogen, and most often, and sulfur. Proteins are found in every part of a living cell and serve as the binding and structural components of all living things, 8, 9

Proximal, toward the point of attachment to the body, 2

Pulmonary circulation, 100, 101

Pulmonary semilunar valve, lets blood travel from the right ventricle into the pulmonary artery and then into the lungs, 99

Pulmonary ventilation, 125–26

Pulmones. See Lungs

Pulse, is an alternating expansion and contraction of the artery as blood flows through it, 104

R

RDA (Recommended Daily Allowance), 139, 141

Red blood cells, contain the red pigment hemoglobin, which is composed of protein and iron. Hemoglobin is vital to the function of the red blood cell as it helps transport oxygen to the tissues and carbon dioxide away from them, 106

Reflex act, is unconscious and involuntary, the simplest type of nerve response, 165

Reproductive system, reproduces human beings, 21

Respiration

cellular, is a chemical process within the cells by which oxygen is used to release energy that is stored in nutrient molecules, such as glucose, 122

external, is the exchange of oxygen and carbon dioxide between the body and the outside environment, 121

internal, involves the exchange of carbon dioxide and oxygen between cells and the surrounding lymph and oxidative process of energy in the cells, 122

Respiratory movements, are the rhythmic movements of the rib cage while air is drawn in and expelled from the lungs, 125–26

Respiratory system, acquires oxygen; rids body of carbon dioxide, 21

is composed of organs that bring oxygen into the body and remove carbon dioxide through a three–stage process identified as external, internal, and cellular respiration, 121

breathing, mechanics of, 125–26

disorders of, 126–28

organs/structures of, 122–24

Reticular layer, is thicker with densely packed with fiber bundles oriented horizontally, rather than vertically as in the papillary layer, and containing fat cells, blood and lymph vessels, oil and sweat glands, hair follicles, and arrector pili, 25

Reticulin, a fibrous protein that works with collagen and elastin to give the dermis elasticity, resilience, and strength, 28

RH blood factor, 107

Rheumatic heart disease, is an infection of the membrane lining the heart, most often caused by streptococci bacteria, that alters heart tissue and affects the valves, causing heart damage, 109

Rheumatoid arthritis, is a chronic systemic disease affecting the connective tissue and joints, 69

Ribs, 64, 66

Rickets, a disease of the bones caused by a lack of vitamin D, calcium, and phosphorous, whereby portions of the bone become soft due to lack of calcification, causing such deformities as bowlegs and knock-knees, 70

S

Sagittal, toward the midline plane of the body, 2

St. Vitus' Dance, is a nervous system disorder that frequently appears following a streptococcal infection, 166

Salt bonds, occur between polypeptide chains, but are not as important as sulphur and hydrogen bonds, except in the case of an unusual reaction to chemical treatment of the hair, 49

Scalp

massage, 83, 85

procedure, 87

Scoliosis, a lateral (horizontal) curvature of the spine, 70

Sebaceous glands, secrete a thick, oily substance known as sebum which lubricates the skin, maintaining its softness and pliability, 27

Secondary hair, 38

Semilunar valves, permit the blood to flow in only one direction, prohibiting it from flowing backward into the chambers, 98

Sense organs, disorders of, 167

Sensory neuron, emerge from the skin or sense organs to send impulses toward the spinal cord and brain, 163

Serum hepatitis, is an inflammation of the liver caused by a virus found only in the blood. It may be transmitted by a blood transfusion contaminated with the virus or through the use of inadequately sterilized needles or surgical equipment, 144

Sex glands, are responsible for fertility and reproduction in both sexes, 158

disorders of, 160

Shingles, is an acute viral nerve infection that is characterized by a one–sided inflammation of cutaneous nerves and which may spread to other nerves, 166

Shoulder girdle, 66

Sickle cell anemia, is a chronic blood disease, inherited from both parents, that causes red blood cells to form in an abnormal shape, 111

Sinusitis, is an infection of the mucous membranes accompanied by pain and nasal discharge, 127

Skeletal system, gives shape to body; protects delicate parts of body; provides space for attaching muscles; is instrumental in forming blood; stores minerals, 21

appendicular, 66–68

axial, 63–65

bones

disorders of, 69–70

structure/formation of, 61–63

types of, 59

joints of, 59–61

motion of, 61

Skin

appendages of, 26–28

bacteria and, 28
massage and, 88
structures of, 23–26
Skull, views of, 65
Sphygmomanometer, a blood pressure–measuring device, 103
Spina bifida, a congenital condition in which the vertebral column does not develop completely and unite correctly, usually affecting the lumbar and sacral regions, 70
Spinal cord, functions as a reflex center and as a pathway to and from the brain, 165
Spine, is strong and flexible, providing support for the head and point of attachment for the head and point attachment for the ribs, 63
view of, 66
Splanchnology, collective study of the digestive, respiratory, reproductive, and urinary systems, 2
Spleen, is a mass of lymphatic tissue that forms lymphocytes and monocytes, filters blood, stores large amounts of red blood cells, forces red blood cells into the circulation when needed, and removes old red blood cells, 108
Sprain, an injury to a joint caused by a sudden or unusual motion, 69
Sternum, 64, 66
Stratum corneum, forms the body's first line of defense against the invasion of bacteria, due to its slightly acidic properties, which can destroy many types of organisms on contact, 25
Stratum germinativum, is an extremely important epidermal layer, as the replacement of cells in the epidermis depends on the division and growth of cells in this layer, 24
Stratum granulosum, consists of cells that look like granules, are almost dead, and have undergone a change into a horny substance, 24
Stratum lucidum, consists of small transparent cells through which light can pass, 24
Sty, is an abscess at the base of an eyelash that is due to the inflammation of a sebaceous gland of the eyelid, 167
Subluxation, one of the most common conditions associated with neck injuries, in which a vertebra is displaced form its normal position or range of motion without being completely dislocated, 70
Sudoriferous glands, 42, 43
apocrine, empty into the canal of the follicle at the point above the sebaceous duct in the armpit, 27
eccrine, open directly onto the surface of the skin, where they secrete large amounts

of diluted salt water when stimulated by heat or emotional stress, 27
Sulphur bonds, join the chains of peptide bonds together horizontally, like rungs of a ladder, 48
Superficial, on or near the surface, 2
Superior
head end of the body (refers to direction), 2
upper, or above another, 2
Sweat glands. See Sudoriferous glands
Synovial fluid, a lubricating substance which reduces the friction of joint movement, 60
Systemic anatomy, is the study of the structure and function of various organs or parts making up a particular organ system, 1
Systolic blood pressure, is the pressure at the moment of the heart muscle's contraction, which is caused by the rush of blood that follows ventricle contractions, 103

T

Tachycardia, is an abnormally rapid heartbeat of 100 beats or more per minute, 110
Tachypnea, is an abnormal rapid rate of shallow breathing, 126
Telogen, keratin formation and, 51
Terminal hair, 38–39
is the long, soft hair found on the scalp, the beard and mustache of adult males, and the legs and underarms of all adults, 37
Tertiary hair, 38–39
is the long, soft hair found on the scalp, the beard and mustache of adult males, and the legs and underarms of all adults, 37
Thalamus, acts as a relay station for incoming and outgoing nerve impulses as it receives direct and/or indirect nerve impulses from various sense organs of the body which are then relayed to the cerebral cortex, 165
Thrombocytes, are the smallest solid components of blood and function in the initial blood–clotting process by producing adhesive structures that stick to collagen fibers in a wound to stop the bleeding, 106
Thrombosis, is a blood clot that forms in a blood vessel or in the heart, 111
Thymus gland
is located in the upper anterior part of the thorax, just above the heart. Its function is to produce lymphocytes, 108
serves as an endocrine gland and as a lymphatic organ until it begins to disappear during puberty, 158

Thyroid cartilage, one of the nine fibrocartilaginous plates which make up the larynx, 122

Thyroid gland, regulates body metabolism and is located on either side of the larynx, where it maintains a rich blood supply, 157–58

Tinnitus, is the sensation of ringing or buzzing in the ear and may be caused by impacted ear wax, otitis media, blockage of normal blood supply, or as a side effect of certain drugs, such as salicylates (pain killers) and quinine, 167

Tissues, 15–23
  are special cells grouped according to function, shape, size, and structures. Tissues form larger functional and structural units known as organs, 4
  burn and, 23
  connective, 17–19
  epithelial, 16–17
  muscle, 20
  nerve, 20
  repair of, 22

Tonsillitis, is an infection of the tonsils, caused by bacteria, that tends to reoccur, 127

Trace elements, needed for health, 140

Trachea, is a tube–like structure, approximately 4 1/2 inches long, that extends from the larynx, passes in front of the esophagus, and continues on to form two bronchi, one for each lung, 124

Tricuspid valve, allows blood flow from the right atrium into the right ventricle, but not in the opposite direction, 99

Trunk, muscles, control breathing and the movements of the abdomen and the pelvis, 76, 78

Tuberculosis, is an infectious disease usually occurring in the lungs, 127

U

Upper extremities, muscles, help move the shoulder (scapula), arm (humerus), forearm, wrist, hand, and fingers, 76, 78

Uremia, is a toxic condition in which the blood retains urinary waste products because the kidneys fail to excrete them, 153

Urinary tract, consisting of two kidneys, two ureters, a bladder, and a urethra, performs the main excretory function of the body, 151–52

V

Varicose veins, is a condition in which the veins break down because of back pressure in the circulatory system, caused by pregnancy or long periods of standing, 88, 102–103

Veins, are less elastic, thinner–walled, and less muscular than arteries, 102
  inflammation of, 88
  valves in, 102
  varicose, is a condition in which the veins break down because of back pressure in the circulatory system, caused by pregnancy or long periods of standing, 88, 102–103

Ventral, in front of, 2

Ventricles, lower chambers of the heart, 98

Vertebrae, are small bones that are separated from each other by pads of cartilage tissue called intervertebral disks, 63

Vertebral column, is strong and flexible, providing support for the head and point of attachment for the ribs, 63
  views of, 66

Virilism, the development of male secondary sex characteristics in a woman, 160

Vitamins, contribute to good health by regulating the metabolism and assisting the biochemical processes that release energy from digested foods, 136
  help the body to control its chemical reactions, 106
  needed in human diet, 138–39
    supplements needed for assimilation of, 137

Voice box, is a triangular chamber located below the pharynx that is composed of nine fibrocartilaginous plates, 122

W

Waste products, elimination of, 142

Waste products, metabolic, are formed by the chemical reactions occurring to maintain homeostasis, 106

Water, digestion and, 135

Whooping cough. See Pertussis

Windpipe, is a tube–like structure, approximately 4 1/2 inches long, that extends from the larynx, passes through the esophagus, and continues on to form two bronchi, one for each lung, 124

Wrist bone, consists of eight small bones arranged in two rows that are held together by ligaments which allow mobility and flexion, 67

Answers to Review Questions

Chapter 1

1. gross anatomy / dermatology
2. Cytology
3. Histology
4. circulatory
5. joints
6. muscular
7. nervous
8. integumentary system / angiology / arthrology / myology / neurology
9. cranial / spinal / thoracic / abdominopelvic
10. dorsal
11. ventral
12. orbital / nasal / buccal
13. massage / steam / pressure / light / environment
14. allergic
15. movement / ingestion / digestion / transport / respiration / synthesis / assimilation / growth / secretion / excretion / regulation / reproduction /
16. energy / food
17. Tissues
18. organs
19. chemical reactions
20. anabolism / catabolism
21. Organs
22. cells / tissues / organs / systems
23. solid / liquid / gas
24. Elements
25. carbon / hydrogen / oxygen / nitrogen
26. Compounds
27. Molecules
28. organic / inorganic
29. carbon
30. Organic
31. carbon / hydrogen / oxygen
32. Monosaccharides
33. Glucose / fructose / galactose
34. table sugar / malt sugar / milk sugar
35. living organisms
36. starch / cellulose / glycogen
37. less
38. Proteins
39. amino acids
40. nine
41. chemical reactions
42. DNA / RNA
43. acid
44. hydroxide ions
45. salt
46. potential hydrogen
47. acidity / alkalinity
48. 0 / 14
49. equal / neutral
50. buffer
51. Amino acids / nucleic acids
52. cell
53. cytoplasm
54. protein synthesis / cell respiration
55. nucleus
56. activities / cell division
57. mitosis
58. cell membrane
59. heat energy
60. Osmosis
61. Filtration
62. nerve cell / red blood cell
63-1. Smooth endoplasmic reticulum
63-2. Ribosomes
63-3. Nucleolus
63-4. Nucleus
63-5. Rough endoplasmic reticulum
63-6. Cell membrane
63-7. Cytoplasm
63-8. Mitochondrion
63-9. Lysosomes
63-10. Chromatin
63-11. Golgi apparatus
63-12. Pinocytic vessel
63-13. Vacuole
64. epithelial / connective / muscle / nerve
65. Epithelial
66. Connective
67. cardiac / striated / nonstriated
68. organ
69. organ system
70. skeletal / muscular / digestive / respiratory / circulatory / reproductive / excretory / endocrine / nervous / integumentary
71. Muscular
72. Digestive
73. Circulatory

74. Skeletal
75. Respiratory
76. Nervous
77. Excretory
78. Integumentary
79. Endocrine
80. Reproductive
81. primary / secondary
82. minor burns / cuts / scrapes
83. cold water
84. dehydration / injury / germ invasion
85. regulation
86. waste
87. fats / glucose / water / salts
88. skin
89. drugs / chemical substances
90. epidermis / dermis
91. stratum corneum / stratum lucidum / stratum granulosum / stratum germinativum
92. Keratin
93. stratum germinativum
94. stratum germinativum / papillary
95. ultraviolet light
96. papillary / reticular
97. papillary
98. reticular
99. subcutaneous tissue
100. seventy
101. collagen
102. Elastin
103. hair / nails / sweat / oil glands / ducts
104. keratinized
105. matrix
106. apocrine / eccrine
107. Apocrine
108. Eccrine
109. emotional stress
110. heat / emotional stress
111. nervous
112. sebum
113. lubricates
114. microbes
115. seven / eight

Chapter 2

1. professionals who perform hair services and treatments on a daily basis
2-1.   scalp treatments
2-2.   massage
3. small downgrowths
4. primary hair
5. secondary hair
6. Tertiary / terminal
7-1.   length
7-2.   texture
8-1.   genetic factors
8-2.   age
8-3.   hormones
8-4.   hormone imbalances
9-1.   S
9-2.   P
9-3   S
9-4   T
9-5   T
9-6   P
9-7   S
9-8   P
9-9   T
9-10   P
9-11   S
9-12   T
9-13   S
9-14   T
9-15   T
9-16   T
10. hair follicle
11. external root / internal root
12. epidermis
13. stratum germinativum
14. columnar cells / cell division
15. matrix
16. internal root sheath
17. hair / external root sheath
18-1.   Hair shaft
18-2.   Stratum corneum
18-3.   Stratum lucidum
18-4.   Stratum granulosum
18-5.   Stratum mucosum
18-6.   Stratum germinativum
18-7.   Papillary layer of dermis
18-8.   Sebaceous (oil) duct
18-9.   Seaceous (oil) gland
18-10.   Arrector pili muscle
18-11.   Capllaries
18-12.   Reticular layer of dermis
18-13.   Papilla of hair
18-14.   Adipose (fatty) tissue
18-15.   Arteries
18-16.   Veins
18-17.   Epidermic scales
18-18.   Sweat pore
18-19.   Epidermis
18-20.   Tactile corpuscle
18-21.   Cold ending
18-22.   Heat ending
18-23.   Touch ending
18-24.   Hair follicle
18-25.   Dermis
18-26.   Sensory nerves
18-27.   Sudoriferous (sweat) duct
18-28.   Sudoriferous (sweat) gland
18-29.   Subcutaneous tissue
18-30.   Pressure ending
18-31.   Sympathetic nerves
19. two / five
20. compound hairs
21. hair bulb / papilla
22. hair bulb
23. papilla
24. keratin
25-1.   fats
25-2.   cholesterol

25-3.   proteins
25-4.   inorganic salts
26. melanin / oxidized oil
27. water / salts / urea / uric acid / amino acids / ammonia / sugar / lactic acid / ascorbic acid
28. Amino acids
29. cortex / injury
30. cortex
31-1.   strength
31-2.   elasticity
31-3.   pliability
31-4.   direction of growth
31-5.   size (or diameter)
31-6.   texture
31-7.   color
31-8.   wave
32. Hydrogen / sulphur bonds
33. physical properties
34. genetic / hereditary
35. number of fibers
36A-1. cuticle
36A-2. cortex
36B-1. 1
36B-2. 2
36B-3. 2
36B-4. 1
36B-5. 1
36B-6. 2
36B-7. 2
36B-8. 1
36B-9. 1
36B-10. 2
37. medulla
38. soft keratin
39-1.   carbon
39-2.   hydrogen
39-3.   oxygen
39-4.   nitrogen
40-1.   simple
40-2.   complex
40-3.   fiber
41. end-bonds / peptide bonds
42. polypeptides
43. Complex proteins

44. Cystine / sulphur bonds
45. Fiber proteins
46-1.   human hair
46-2.   animal hair
46-3.   silk
46-4.   horn of some animals
47. sulphur
48. Hair
49. Peptide bonds
50. Sulphur / cystine bonds
51. cystine / disulfide bonds
52. tensile strength
53. cysteine
54. neutralizing
55-1.   ammonium thioglycolate
55-2.   sodium hydroxide
56-1.   neutralizer
56-2.   hydrogen peroxide
56-3.   oxygen
57. numerous
58. hydrogen bonds
59. physical bonds
60-1.   water
60-2.   dilute alkali
60-3.   neutral lotions
60-4.   acid lotions
61-1.   air drying
61-2.   dilute acids
62. between the chains of keratin
63. Free amino acids
64. Salt, carbon / nitrogen
65. anagen / catagen / telogen
66. germinativa / keratinization
67. follicle
68. catagen
69. papilla / hair bulb
70. telogen

Chapter 3

1. 206

2. support / body structures / shape / internal organs / movement / anchorage / mineral / blood cell
3. long / short / irregular / flat
4. Joints
5. bone shape / joint
6. degree / movement
7. diarthroses
8. cartilage
9. Synovial fluid
10. ossified / arthritis
11. shoulders or hips
12. knees, elbows, or outer joints of fingers
13. forearm
14. vertebrae
15. Ligaments
16. Tendons
17. Flexion
18. Extension
19. rotation
20. 35 percent organic / 65 percent inorganic
21. bone collagen
22. mineral salts
23. white blood
24. red blood
25. center / ends
26. axial / appendicular
27. cranial / facial
28. eight / fourteen
29. mucous membranes
30. Colds / hayfever / allergies
31. encloses / protects
32. proper balance
33. twelve
34. clavicles
35. arm
36. humerus
37. radius
38. rotate
39. eight
40. 5 metacarpal / 14 phalanges

41. seven
42. five
43. Arches
44. weight
45. client consultation / observation
46. Pain
47. Fractures / breaks
48. Massage
49. amphiarthroses
50. synarthroses
51. diarthroses
52. Dislocation
53. Closed fracture
54. Arthritis
55. Gouty arthritis
56. Sprain
57. Rheumatoid arthritis
58. Osteoporosis
59. Bursitis

Chapter 4

1. contractibility
2. half
3. move / erect / influences posture / body heat / internal organs / form
4. skeletal / smooth / cardiac
5. Voluntary
6. Involuntary
6. Involuntary
8. contractibility / extensibility / elasticity
9. tendons
10. origin
11. insertion
12. belly
13. pairs
14. opposite
15. lactic acid
16. Muscle tone
17. facial expression / mastication
18. extension / flexion / rotation
19. upper extremities
20. trunk
21. lower extremities
22. size, / structure / strength
23. physical
24. light / heat / cold / water / electricity / massage / exercise
25. Muscular tissue
26. Therapeutic
27. flat feet, muscle hypertrophy, muscle fatigue, stiff neck / muscle spasms
28. exercise, good nutrition, good posture / regular massage.
29. Massage
30. body temperature is over 99.4 degrees Fahrenheit
31. an acute infectious disease is present
32. an inflamed area may be further irritated
33. varicose veins are present
34. edema is present
35. the client has high blood pressure
36. the client is intoxicated
37. Deep pressure
38. soothing / relaxing
39. six
40. Petrissage
41. Vibration
42. Effleurage
43. Friction
44. Percussion

Chapter 5

1. closed circulatory
2. liquid
3. plasma / liquid / blood cells / solid
4. red blood / white blood / platelets
5. oxygen / carbon dioxide
6. White blood
7. Platelets
8. suspends / transports
9. nutritive / respiratory / excretory / regulatory / protective
10. heart
11. lymphatic
12. general / pulmonary
13. to
14. from / lungs
15. muscle
16. Cardiopulmonary resuscitation
17. 75
18. deoxygenated
19. oxygenated
20. four
21. atria
22. ventricles
23. Valves
24. heart muscle
25. electrical
26. Atrial / ventricle
27. cardiac cycle
28. aorta
29. ascending
30. descending
31. lungs
32. away from / venules
33. Capillaries
34. Nutrient / oxygen, / metabolic
35. varicose veins
36. Systolic
37. highest
38. diastolic
39. sphygmomanometer
40. systolic / diastolic
41. 120/80
42. heart attacks / strokes
43. steam towel facials / full-body massages / body wraps / tanning booths

44. pulse
45. 78 / 80
46. protein
47. blood clotting
48. chemical / acid-base
49. Hormones / vitamins / enzymes
50. erythrocytes
51. leukocytes
52. chemical damage / physical trauma / pathogenic
53. redness / local heat / swelling / pain
54. Pus
55. four / six
56. inherited
57. agglutinogen
58. A / B / AB / O
59. Individually
60. Individually
61. Jointly
62. Not at all
63. circulatory
64. lymphatic
65. capillaries / tissues
66. food / oxygen / hormones
67. away from
68. blood vessels
69. lymphatic production / filter
70. Natural immunity
71. Acquired immunity
72. passive / active
73. artificial
74. hypersensitivity
75. allergic
76. allergic reaction
77. Cardiovascular
78. Streptococci
79. arrhythmia
80. arterial fibrillation
81. heart failure
82. angina pectoris
83. vein
84. anemia
85. iron

86. embolism
87. hereditary
88. over
89. acquired immune deficiency syndrome
90. disorder
91. human immunodeficiency virus / HIV
92. C
93. D
94. B
95. A
96. c
97. d
98. b
99. a
100. b
101. d
102. b
103. c
104. opportunistic
105. two / six
106. seroconversion
107. immune
108. stimulate

Chapter 6

1. oxygen / carbon dioxide
2. external / internal / cellular
3. Int
4. C
5. Ex
6. Ex
7. Int
8. Ex
9. C
10. Air / lungs
11. filter
12. mucus / blood vessels
13. mucous
14. Nerve endings
15. resonance / voice
16. larynx
17. thyroid / Adam's apple
18. vocal cords

19. relaxed / low
20. tense / high
21. two
22. trachea
23. C-shaped rings
24. abdominal thrust
25. aveoli / capillaries
26. red blood cells
27. Oxygen
28. apex
29. Air
30. three / two
31. friction
32. pressure changes
33. cellular respiration / mechanical
34. inhalation
35. Internal
36. one
37. 14 / 20
38. Respiratory rate
39. Nervous / chemical
40. brain stem
41. involuntary
42. reflex
43. carbon dioxide
44. rate / sound
45. virus
46. bacteria / viruses / irritants
47. pharyngitis
48. Laryngitis
49. bacteria
50. mucous membranes
51. Bronchitis
52. irritating vapors
53. Pneumonia
54. organ / tissue
55. infectious
56. whooping cough
57. emotion / stress / breathing / irritants
58. overinflation
59. cancer
60. D
61. F
62. A
63. B

64. C
65. E
66. G

Chapter 7

1. physical / chemical
2. simple soluble
3. Enzymatic hydrolysis
4. enzymes
5. chemical changes
6. not
7. alimentary / accessory
8. digestive / gastrointestinal
9. ali
10. acc
11. acc
12. ali
13. acc
14. ali
15. ali
16. ali
17. ali
18. ali
19. digested
20. mechanically
21. Saliva
22. small
23. bloodstream
24. energy / repair / production
25. large
26. liver bile / pancreatic juice
27. fat
28. protein / starch / fat
29. bile
30. Water
31. nonpathogenic
32. acids / gases / waste products
33. B-complex / K
34. Vitamin K
35. water / carbohydrates / lipids / proteins / minerals / vitamins
36. water

37. 55 / 65
38. food
39. carbohydrates
40. energy / minerals / vitamins / roughage
41. Lipids
42. fats
43. vitamin D
44. arterial plaque
45. hormones / enzymes / genes
46. amino acids
47. combination
48. transmitters
49. vitamins / minerals
50. complex
51. vitamin B-12
52. metabolism / biochemical
53. micronutrients
54. water / oil
55. C / B-complex
56. synergy
57. Enzymes
58. specific function
59. coenzymes
60. body fluids
61. minerals
62. nerve
63. inorganic
64. antioxidants
65. atoms
66. minimum
67. chemical
68. organically grown
69. heat
70. Frozen
71. high blood pressure / heart disease / stroke
72. circulate
73. gland
74. Hypoglycemia
75. Complex
76. chloride
77. antacids / pain / inflammation
78. nerve cells
79. Obesity

80. sensitivity / allergies
81. psychologically
82. Bulimia
83. diet / nutrition
84. C
85. D
86. B
87. E
88. A
89. H
90. I
91. J
92. K
93. L
94. G
95. F

Chapter 8

1. digestible / undigestible
2. toxins
3. kidneys / skin / intestines / lungs
4. carbon dioxide / water vapor
5. urinary system
6. perspiration
7. intestines
8. excretory
9. Urine
10. blood pressure
11. useful / water
12. osmosis
13. antidiuretic
14. opposite
15. blood
16. reservoir
17. nervous
18. acute kidney failure
19. bacterial
20. incontinence
21. Kidney stones

Chapter 9

1. specific
2. gland

3. ductless
4. hormones
5. directly
6. pituitary
7. master
8. Pituitary
9. pituitary
10. starch / sugar
11. metabolism
12. thyroid
13. blood clotting
14. disappears
15. anti-inflammatory
16. Corticoids
17. fertility / reproduction
18. internal / external
19. Insulin
20. Endocrine disorders
21. hyperactivity / hypoactivity
22. thyroid
23. Hyperthyroidism
24. underactive
25. pituitary
26. dwarfism
27. male
28. electrolytes
29. Pancreatic
30. C
31. D
32. B
33. E
34. F
35. A

Chapter 10

1. endocrine / nervous

2. brain / spinal cord / nerves
3. communicate
4. sensory / motor / connecting.
5. Sensory
6. sensory
7. Motor
8. neuron
9. three
10. involuntary / glands
11. decision / action
12. nervous
13-a. acts as a shock absorber for the brain and spinal cord
13-b. transports nutrients to the brain cells
13-c. removes waste products from the brain cells
14. cerebrum / cerebellum / brain stem
15. cerebrum
16. two
17. four
18. functions
19. frontal
20. parietal
21. occipital
22. temporal
23-a. conscious thought
23-b. judgment
23-c. reasoning
23-d. memory
23-e. will power
24. thalamus
25-a. autonomic nervous control

25-b. cardiovascular control
25-c. temperature control
25-d. appetite control
25-e. water balance
25-f. emotional state
25-g. gastrointestinal control
25-h. sleep control
26. cerebellum
27. impaired
28. midbrain / pons / medulla
29. respiration
30. pons
31. midbrain
32. sleep / moods
33. medulla
34. medulla
35. reflex
36. reflex act
37. stimulus
38. Chorea
39. herpes zoster
40. viral
41. infectious
42. encephalitis
43. Convulsions
44. meningitis
45. Epilepsy
46. otitis
47. Tinnitus
48. Conjunctivitis
49. sty
50. Glaucoma
51. cataract
52. C
53. A
54. B